primary care

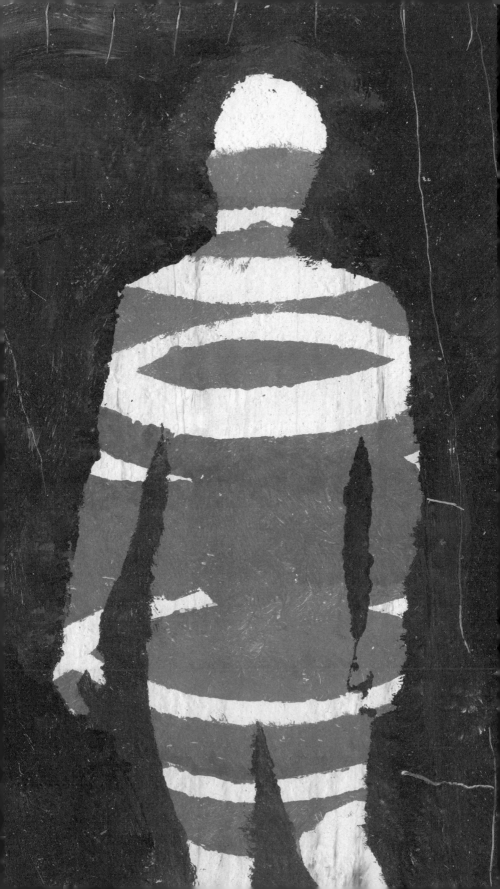

MORE POEMS BY PHYSICIANS

primary care

edited by ANGELA BELLI and JACK COULEHAN

University of Iowa Press IOWA CITY

University of Iowa Press,
Iowa City 52242
http://www.uiowapress.org
Copyright © 2006 by
the University of Iowa Press

The University of Iowa Press is a
member of Green Press Initiative and
is committed to preserving natural
resources.

Printed on acid-free paper

Library of Congress
Cataloging-in-Publication Data
Primary care: more poems by physicians /
edited by Angela Belli and Jack Coulehan.
p. cm.
ISBN-13: 978-1-58729-502-7 (cloth)
ISBN-10: 1-58729-502-4 (cloth)
ISBN-13: 978-1-58729-503-4 (pbk.)
ISBN-10: 1-58729-503-2 (pbk.)
1. Physicians' writings, American.
2. American poetry—21st century.
3. Body, Human—Poetry.
4. Physicians—Poetry.   5. Medicine—
Poetry.   I. Belli, Angela.   II. Coulehan,
John L. (Jack), 1943–.
PS591.P48P75 2006
811'.5408356—dc22   2006044563

06 07 08 09 10 C 5 4 3 2 1
06 07 08 09 10 P 5 4 3 2 1

CONTENTS

INTRODUCTION

When Americans speak about their health care, the stories they tell are often contradictory and confusing. Americans are justly proud of our great hospitals with their immense technological arsenals: laser surgery, colonoscopy, positron emission tomography, mini-laparoscopies, implantable defibrillators, powerful chemotherapy, and the list continues on and on. Our present metaphor in medicine is war and aggression; we fight disease relentlessly, often no matter what the cost, and sometimes without considering very carefully how much suffering or collateral damage the battle will entail. Because of its spectacular success in so many areas, health care plays an ever increasing role in our culture, to the extent that 16 percent of our Gross Domestic Product is devoted to health care. Americans routinely expect medical miracles. They believe that at least some effective treatment can be provided for any disease, if only you find the right hospital or specialist. If treatment isn't effective, something must be wrong.

Americans also tell a second type of story, and they do so with greater and greater frequency. These stories are full of anger and disillusionment, skepticism and pain. In part, they confirm health care studies and international comparisons. For example, consider the high prevalence of medical mistakes; the 46 million Americans who can't afford health insurance; and the fact that the United States falls behind many other countries in indices of medical outcomes and public health. We rank fiftieth among the world's countries in infant mortality and twenty-fourth in life expectancy. Most remarkably, studies show that the majority of Americans express dissatisfaction with their health care system.

However, these statistical findings are merely illustrative. The real stories arise from people's personal experiences as they negotiate their way through the complex and daunting health care bureaucracy. It almost seems a matter of astrology, where the various planets—health insurance, type of illness, physician availability, and personal assertiveness—have to be in proper conjunction before the patient has a chance at obtaining a prompt appointment and an attentive and sympathetic hearing. The key word in the previous sentence is "attentive." The majority of personal stories about medical interactions include statements like the following: "My doctor doesn't listen to me," "She's always in too much of a hurry," and "He has his own agenda—he doesn't want to hear what I'm saying."

In other words, these patients experience their physicians as not taking their stories seriously or not being carefully attentive to them as persons, as subjects, rather than merely as objects that happen to harbor a disease. If this is true, these physicians are not exhibiting the quality and skill called clinical empathy, the skill that helps physicians understand what the patient is actually experiencing and, thereby, creates a connection of trust and respect between the two parties. More-over, in many of these stories, patients speak with anxiety and confusion about their doctors' use of language: "She used words that I couldn't understand," or "He told me I had a time bomb in my chest; now I'm scared to death." The same physicians who fail to listen also fail to understand the power of language to heal—*and* to harm, as in the preceding example.

This is where poetry enters the scene. It doesn't necessarily come galloping in on a white horse, because there are many other methods for physicians to learn to enhance their attentiveness, empathy, and respect for language. Nonetheless, poetry—as language, rhythm, image, metaphor, and symbol—lies at the core of cultural healing traditions throughout the world. We suspect that most people, upon hearing that in many American medical schools students are being taught poetry, would be incredulous. They would similarly be surprised to discover that the tradition linking healing and poetry is not alien to American soil, having gained entry at Rutherford, New Jersey, through the art of physician-poet William Carlos Williams. Separated from Williams by a full generation and half a conti-nent, Iowa poet Paul Engle paid homage to Williams in a piece contrasting his life on the midwestern prairie to that of Williams in industrial New Jersey. What linked them was a shared dedication to the wonders of poetry. Fittingly, Engle defined Williams's gift in his own verse, "Like the antibiotics he learned to use, his poems / heal and are healthy."[1]

Such truth aside, most people would also find it peculiar that medical students are learning how to write and analyze personal narratives and meeting regularly with their peers to share uncertainties, emotions, and ambivalence that arise in their professional relationships. Finally, our representatives of the high-tech, machine-addicted culture would be absolutely astounded that patients who suf-fer from chronic illnesses often begin to function better and obtain symptomatic relief by writing poetry themselves.

The poetry movement in medicine is, in one sense, self-consciously instru-mental. We teach poetry to help students enhance their empathy, to understand what aging, or dying, or bereavement, or childbirth, or mental illness, or cultural alienation feels like. In this instrumental context, poetry sometimes breaks through a seemingly impenetrable barrier. It's not easy. When faced with a poetry assignment, students immediately complain: "Aw, don't ask us to read poetry." "I can't understand it." "It's too complicated." "Poetry doesn't have anything to do with medicine." "I just can't see the point." "It doesn't have a point."

"*Anything* but poetry!"

Yet, surprisingly, when they are forced (perhaps that is too strong a word) to drop preconceived notions and set their anxiety aside, the subsequent discussion is often extraordinarily energizing because once having entered into the poem they feel free to speak from their hearts, rather than being chained to the left side of their brains, which is usually the situation in medical school. Of course, for poetry to have this effect, it has to be honest and direct, as opposed to allusive and obscure, characteristics that many Americans associate with poetry when they say, "I just can't understand it."

However, there is a sense in which the poetry movement in medical schools is pulled from above, rather than pushed from below. Medicine has always been an emotionally and spiritually challenging profession. Nowadays, confronted with the rapid progress of technology, the shifting sands of health care economics and glaring disparities in health care and human rights in our Global Village, physicians experience challenges that grow constantly more demanding. Many physicians attempt to build into their lives opportunities for reflection and self-awareness. It is in this context that medical poetry has blossomed. We use the word "blossomed" with confidence, surely in terms of quality and probably also in quantity, although we lack data on the number of poets per thousand physicians. In the last twenty-five years the number of medical venues featuring poetry has increased dramatically. Nowadays most major general medical journals publish poems regularly, usually in conjunction with other narrative features, like short stories and personal essays. Some specialty journals also present poetry and other creative writing. Moreover, numerous physician-poets publish their work in literary magazines and produce full-length collections, some of which have won substantial literary awards. Likewise, several poetry anthologies have appeared, either consisting entirely of poetry written by physicians (The Naked Physician, Blood and Bone, On Being a Doctor) or of works related to health care that include works by physicians (Uncharted Lines, Articulations). Finally, in 2004 the first large scale poetry and medicine conference was held at Duke University, featuring talks and workshops by leading American poets like Lucille Clifton, Sharon Olds, Alan Shapiro, and Mark Doty and well-known physician-poets such as John Stone and Rafael Campo.

The poets whose work is sampled in this collection are representative of physicians who utilize the language of poetry as a means of personal reflection and self-expression. Thus, when we ask students to write poetry in order to help them to reflect upon their experiences of the treacherous, emotionally charged world of medical training, these poets can truly be called their mentors: doctors who are walking the walk, as well as talking the talk, who are facing (or have faced) a life in medicine and developed a peculiarly medical way of looking at the world, a medical sensibility.

For the last fifty years or so, medical educators have used terms like detachment, objectivity, and detached concern to characterize the physicians' proper relationship to his or her patient. Often these educators interpreted *aequanimitas*, a Latin term employed by the iconic physician and educator Sir William Osler in his writings about professionalism, to mean detachment and self-possession, thus suggesting that the early-twentieth-century Osler was urging doctors to distance themselves from their patients, as is the common "wisdom" of today.[2] However, a more accurate, and in the context of Osler's life a more appropriate, interpretation of *aequanimitas* refers to the physician's inner calmness and tolerance, as opposed to detachment or coldness. We sometimes borrow the words *steadiness* and *tenderness* from Thomas Percival, the eighteenth-century physician who published the first modern book of medical ethics in 1803. Percival enjoined physicians to "unite tenderness with steadiness" in their care of patients. This union, or perhaps "dynamic tension" is a better term, is the basis for good doctoring and, we believe, of a medical sensibility that frequently informs the creative writing of physicians. Percival contrasts "coldness of heart," which often develops in practitioners who cultivate emotional detachment, with the "tender charity" that the moral practice of medicine requires: "This coldness of heart, this moral insensibility, should be sedulously counteracted before it has gained an invincible ascendancy."[3]

If asked why they write, the poets represented in this anthology would likely give reasons similar to those of other poets. To them it feels natural to make poems; they experience a need to express themselves in this way. This would have been the case had they become attorneys, business executives, or forest rangers, rather than physicians. Nonetheless, doctoring provides poets with unusually broad and deep access to human suffering, as well as tenacity, heroism, love, and joy. It also puts the practitioner at risk of coldness of heart, a risk that all share, but which goes with the territory in medicine. Quite naturally, a rather high percentage of the poems in this collection arise from the physician's life at work—with the uncertainty, pain, anger, sympathy, longing, skepticism, desperation, and love they observe in their patients, and often experience themselves. In addition, physician-poets often write of private concerns; they acquaint us with members of their families and share confidences regarding personal relationships; and they exhibit a social consciousness that is meaningful for us all as citizens of one nation and of one world.

A preview of the collection provides a glimpse of the rich and diverse content that awaits the reader.

It is not uncommon to find physicians sharing their patients' feelings even as they share their apprehensions regarding the state of their own health. As patients acquire the medical facts about themselves via ever-advancing technological means, they must face a common side effect—the realization that their daily lives may very well be altered, for good or ill, by the knowledge gained. The physician, too, may have a similar awareness in confronting the facts when confirmed in like manner. In "My Tomography Report" John Wright records the tension between certainty and disquiet that he deals with daily as a consequence of new knowledge. Unlike the physician, the patient's pursuit of the facts often reflects the fantasy that successful treatment is attainable for any disorder so long as one finds the proper physician who commands the necessary knowledge. Dannie Abse gives such a patient a voice and transmits the unreasoned belief in "Among a Heap of Stones." Marc J. Straus provides the answer for Abse in "Not God," although the patient who asks hard questions of him allows his physician a margin of fallibility. Straus concedes that he is not God. But his reply is tinged with doubt.

Technology cannot always provide the answers that physicians and patients seek. In Shen's "Two Men" the husband of a dying woman questions the physician at her side. The answer sought, inadequate to soothe his pain, is suspended as a buzzing morphine pump provides an easy answer to the wife's pain. The need to acknowledge "when it's over" is advice given in Bonnie Salomon's "Call It." The call is not an admission of defeat but a recognition that when an event, be it a life or a ball game, reaches its conclusion, little remains but to accept the finality of the experience. The call may be made with confidence when nothing has been neglected that could alter the outcome. When, on occasion, matters are handled with less than scrupulous attention, grievous consequences may result. Consider the situation in which Audrey Shafer finds herself in "Incompatibility" when the incredulous physician must confront the fact that during surgery her patient was given blood incompatible with his own. The operating room becomes the locus of a struggle to counter the pernicious effects of the mistake. The routine of a physician's day at work is sadly punctured in Richard Berlin's "Piano Music" when the call comes unexpectedly for a colleague and friend. On the day that would be his last, the physician took time from a busy schedule to confide in the poet a wish to learn to play the piano. The shock of his sudden death resounds throughout the hospital. The music that remains is the verse that holds him in memory.

The workplace itself is often a subject of examination. In Saxby Pridmore's "New Secure Psychiatric Unit" the speaker scans a unit without patients. Designers have decorated the new facility with care. For the moment it stands untarnished—awaiting the time when it will be populated by suffering occupants, grieving parents, and vigilant critics. In Iain Bamforth's "A Shining" the workplace extends to the wilderness, to the rural farmhouse of a family whose peace the physician must disrupt by the delivery of bad news. By contrast, the tranquility of another home visited by Beth Lown in "Home Visit" remains. Leaving the busy hospital, the poet rushes to keep an appointment with an elderly couple. As she stands by their door, she catches sight of the slumbering pair through a window and pauses, hesitant to ring the bell that will disturb their rest. Daniel C.

Bryant visits his patients in a nursing facility and finds them less than hospitable in "Nursing Home." In fact, they withdraw from him. Many prefer the company of handsome soldiers in faded photographs. John Stone's visit to his mother in the home where she resides in "Visitation" captures a tender moment when her son shows the aged woman a photograph of his long-deceased father. Studying her husband's face, his widow has no memory of him. But she still finds him handsome. The photograph that the patient shows his visitor in Craig Powell's "Poem (Long Overdue) for Mr. Meek" is of his wife who died some years before. The likeness endures despite being nibbled on by rats. The patient, too, endures despite the small agonies of his daily existence.

Physicians are often foregrounded in these poems. Taken together, they comprise a varied roster. While not deified, the physician in Frederic Platt's "Mother Teresa, the Cardiologist" would approach sainthood, were it not for his devotion to a lucrative specialty which subsumes his passion for humanity. The satirical portrait is rounded with the revelation that the subject would ask God for help— not to treat the poor but to improve his golf score. Humanity is of little concern to the iconic figure of Richard Bronson's "Plague Doctor." Venturing out into the plague-stricken city, he visits the victims to confirm their illness, a duty eschewed by the qualified doctors that have fled in fear of becoming themselves contaminated. The poet ponders the obscure motives of the figure dressed in the curious protective gear of his calling, including a doctor's hat and a stick with which to push away the sick that approach him. A doctor in training comes in contact with the infected in David Moolten's "Che Guevara at the San Pablo Leper Colony, 1952." The poem marks moments in the life of the Latin American rebel, most notably Guevara's visit to a camp for lepers in Peru where he greeted the untouchable peasants with his bare hands. The visit significantly influenced both the development of his political credo and the tension between dedicating himself to medicine or to the revolutionary activities that would eventually preoccupy him.

A selection of poems deals with the inglorious but humorous aspects of comedy seen so frequently in medicine. The education of a physician does not often point a direction for a life of political activism. The experience can be stressful enough, but in retrospect one can appreciate its humorous aspects. In "Advice to a First-Year Medical Student" Sharon Balter recalls being taught the value of anticipating every possible need in the performance of her duties. Determined to succeed, she repeats the well-intentioned advice until the lesson dominates her every waking and sleeping moment. The image of the young woman sleeping in her shoes so that she may always be prepared provokes humor while giving rise to sympathy for the dedicated student. In "That Intern Dream" Jack Coulehan similarly recalls the anxieties to which the young and inexperienced are subject in the exercise of a demanding craft. The emotions are recollected in a recurring nightmare of the poet's in which his younger self finds his worst fears realized—caught unprepared in a medical emergency. The intern makes all the wrong decisions in a rapidly deteriorating situation. While the events in the nightmare are terrifying for the young man, and for the dreamer as well, they provide much amusement for the reader.

A sober maturity marks the tone of David Watts's "The Day I Showed My Penis to the Lady Doctor." A physical examination that could prove embarrassing for a male patient and a female doctor is conducted with both participants exhibiting admirable scientific objectivity, with both displaying proper professional detachment, with both reflecting a seasoned awareness of the art of doctoring. At its conclusion, both dash for the door. Humor is frequently used as a means of relieving tension, often enough in medical situations. An attempt to do so by Tim Metcalf in "The Muse Collapses" ends in failure when his patient in distress fails to be comforted by his efforts at gallantry and humor. She ignores his amusing rhyme, leading him to conclude that whatever her condition, it is certain that her blood contains no poetry. The muse suffers a setback.

The laughter engendered in many of these poems results from situations removed from work. In "After the Concert: A Confession" John Stone recalls being seated beside a strange woman at a performance of a Brahms string quartet while they shared the passion of the music. As the fugue reached its climax, the poet simultaneously felt an overwhelming desire to ask the woman to dance. The "punch line" that ends the verse provides the humor. A droll bit of humor emerges from D. A. Feinfeld's "Itch." Compared to pain, the itching sensation deprives one of dignity. Having the back of one's neck tickled with a feather inspires laughter not sympathy. Only the affected can understand why "Old Scratch" is an appropriate nickname for the devil.

The impact of illness upon identity is a subject explored by several of the poets in the collection. Robert Harlan Wintroub is among them. In "Heart Sounds" he reveals the transformation that occurs in a woman who resigns herself to accepting her body as an object of detached scrutiny all the while remembering a past when she viewed herself as an object of sexual desire. Similarly, Alice Jones's "Expunge" depicts a woman who puts aside all thoughts of intimacy following a mastectomy. She disavows the letters from her lover that lie hidden away from her sight and from her mind. Instead, she gives her attention to remedies for her body, her pool, and her old canvases.

A number of poems raise our curiosity about patients who never appear. Peter Goldsworthy's "Suicide on Christmas Eve" sets a holiday scene that is characterized by reflection. The figures in the poem ponder the meaning of existence while one who is absent determines that life is devoid of meaning. The solitary patient who lies dying in the ICU in Dwaine Rieves's "Shifts" is virtually absent from the scene, except as a voice on a telephone answering machine replying to attempts to gather information. The voice that outlives the body offers polite thanks for the call. In contrast, the absence of a voice in a living body points to a disability in Jennifer Harrison's "Aus-Lan." Here the poet learns how the deaf communicate. A disputed issue among the deaf population—the use of sign language as opposed to speech—remains in the background. The reader discovers the value of signing through the poem's imagery that shows the effectiveness of the language of the body in expressing meanings that reach beyond words.

The speaker in Ronald Pies's "The Alzheimer Sonnets" is vocal enough, but his identity is never fixed, undergoing change as he progresses from childhood to maturity in the four sonnets that comprise the work. Much of the past is obscure for the aged patient of the final lines. Yet the soul hunts for instances of experience that validate an entire life. A vivid portrait of an individual who once commanded language yet yielded to the omnipotence of nature is created in George Young's "Emerson's Aphasia." Attempting to gauge the speed of life is a futile exercise, particularly with ordinary means of measurement, as Karl Weyrauch discovers in "My Speedometer." The instrument fails to cope with high speed in an automobile, let alone calculate the pace at which the poet is carried into the future. In "Entitlements" George Braman considers the gradual way in which middle age comes upon one. Caught unaware, the individual experiences a slow but general decline of faculties. The experience is universal.

As to be expected, an interest in human anatomy is everywhere apparent. In Arthur Ginsberg' s "Epithalamium," the brain comes under close scrutiny. Fascinated by the exposed structure in a patient undergoing surgery, the poet searches without success among ridges and ruts to trace the formation of a thought. Agreeing with Ronald Pies, he concludes that the brain must be the bridegroom of the soul. In Jack Coulehan's "Phrenology," the shape of the skull is examined tenderly to provide a clue to character. In the final quatrain the poet observes that locks of hair disguise the bumps on his beloved's skull, making a reading more difficult. As Kirsten Emmott points out in "Anatomy," a woman's character is not easily defined. Even an examination of a woman's body fails to reveal her nature. The fascination that patients maintain for a dysfunctional body part that has been replaced with a reasonable facsimile, particularly a heart, puzzles Paul Boor in "Blood Song" as he notes the rare appearance of individuals at the surgical pathology lab who come to retrieve their extricated organs. The request poses a dilemma: Does one hand it over in a brown paper bag? A jar? And then, he wonders, how would it look on the coffee table?

A good number of poems move well beyond the clinical sphere in dealing with personal matters. Frequently they explore family relationships. Dealing with the death of a brother in "Five Tasks," Patrick Clary gives the man new life as he recreates him in verse and introduces him to the reader who never knew him. The dead man emerges as a vibrant, living presence who is perceived through the power of love fueling an artistic sensibility. In Richard Donzé's "Four Perfect Quarters," the enduring pain of loss is conveyed in images that tell of a relationship between student and teacher. The two bonded in meeting the challenges of nature. The student who survives recalls the deceased teacher each time that he applies his honed skills, wishing only that he could demonstrate to him how well the lessons had been taught. The relationship between the generations concerns poet Robert Carroll in "Show and Tell." A son with a drug dependency causes a horrified father to reflect on the way in which each of us is responsible for the future of all. In "Radiology" Catherine Caldicott reveals the thoughts of a mother awaiting the result of her seven-year-old son's brain scan. As she waits, she offers her own analysis, identifying the areas of his brain that give evidence of his intelligence, independence, drive, and creativity. Fearing the worst, she pleads with the doctor to show her his "giggle cells."

Frequently, it is young patients who dominate the scene in these verses. They are treated with sensitivity and compassion, though they may oppose their physicians and resist treatment. Such is the case in John Graham-Pole's "Health Care," where a thirteen-year-old with a brain tumor vigorously rejects the efforts of those who would help him. He screams curses at them and demands to die while they make frantic efforts to prolong his life. Meanwhile, in an unattended dressing room, an intruder is busily at work burglarizing their valuables. Chuck Joy's patient in "What If Lashika?" is a seventeen-year-old who enjoys the pose of a troublesome adolescent. Her physician imagines what it would be like should Lashika approach him one day with a smile and a cordial greeting. He concludes that life is not long enough for either one to witness such a change. Only if art gives way to life and an actor creates the desired personality can the metamorphosis occur. The thirteen-year-old who is lucky at Monopoly is the cousin of poet Wayne Liebman. Her success at the game of chance—she wins every time they play—is achieved with ease in "Monopoly." Fifteen years later, chance will work against her and she will lose her life as well as that of her infant son in a fatal automobile accident. In "Kindergarten Physical" Kelley Jean White introduces us to a docile, fragile child. A victim of physical abuse, the youngster has scars on his body that are not hidden by his superman underwear. Only a sock conceals the ring around his toe, ever in place for when his mother chains him in the basement. The undeveloped fetus in Peter Pereira's "Fetus Papyraceous" remains a phenomenon. He forfeits his life to his more viable twin whose growth compresses him in utero. All that remains of him is a faint imprint in a web of membranes. The poet wonders if half of the living twin's soul remains shrouded within the paper-thin form of the fetus. The dehumanizing physical anomalies that result from genetic misarrangements raise questions in Thomas Dorsett's "Trisomy 13" about divine wisdom and goodness. It remains to the parents to accept the impaired infant whose human identity is challenged. The troubled offspring of separated parents finds an antidote to loneliness in Elspeth Cameron Ritchie's "Gun in the Closet"; it combines his knowledge of the use of firearms and the location of a gun in the house. Suicide is the option chosen by Joseph Meister, who made medical history as a nine-year-old when he became the first human to be inoculated by Louis Pasteur in a successful treatment for rabies. George Young narrates his tale in "The Face of Evil." Enjoying good health for the remainder of his sixty-four years, Meister repaid his debt to "dear Monsieur Pasteur" in 1940 when, rather than opening the scientist's burial crypt to the Wehrmacht, he went home and shot himself with his World War I service revolver.

A significant number of poems collected herein reveal the poets' social awareness as they focus on local and global issues. An event that is easily absorbed in the daily happenings of a large city is magnified by Serena Fox in "Another Drive-By." Using the traditional form of the sonnet, the poet expresses contemporary experience, relaying the swift pace of city life and the birth of an addicted baby to a drug-dependent mother in the back seat of a cab—between fares. Paramedics rush to give aid as the taxi vanishes into the night. In "Bellevue Hospital Blues" Herbert Krohn traces the progress of New York City's East River as it runs past the nation's oldest public hospital and out to sea. He marks the numberless city dwellers that lived and died in the structure's environs and notes the suicides that drowned in the river. He hears the little moans of infants whose empty cradles lie in the damp cellar of the building.

From the city to the world—a good number of poems deal with issues of concern around the globe. Poets expand their visions to encompass life beyond our shores and to comment on social upheavals caused by human brutality. Because they recognize the power of language to heal (as well as to damage), physician-poets speak out publicly, as poets have always done. With a sensibility that unites steadiness and tenderness, these writers look directly at the injustice and terror of a contemporary world that is increasingly polarized by poverty, politics, fanaticism, and religion. The events of the recent past remain vivid for many. In "Cambodians Celebrate the Buddhist New Year Once Again" Norbert Hirschhorn observes families celebrating a holy day. His thoughts turn to the rituals performed by Jews since biblical times in observance of the High Holy Days. In these rituals or "holocausts," sacrificial sheep were wholly consumed by fire. Michael Lieberman's resolve in "Pledge" is short-lived. He determines not to obsess any longer over the evil perpetrated by the Nazis in the murder of the innocents. He will no longer think of the Holocaust—not until the next day.

More recent events as well are reflected in these pages. In comparing the current collection to our previous anthology of poetry by physicians, *Blood and Bone: Poems by Physicians*, one striking difference is immediately apparent. September 11, 2001, had not yet happened when the previous work appeared. Nowhere is the medical sensibility more in evidence than in the contemplation of the events of that day. And never before has that sensibility been more wounded. Considering the history of medicine and its dedication to relieving suffering and prolonging life over the centuries, together with the ever-renewed oath of its practitioners to do no harm, what response is to be expected from that sphere to the wanton and senseless destruction of life on a grand scale? Contributors to the current collection record their reactions in the poems we come upon here. Holding the victims of the attack in memory, Rafael Campo shares with us his vision in "Questions for the Weather." He views the airplane roaring over the city as signaling the approach of Armageddon. Similarly, Ted McMahon in "9-11" is sensitive to how what may prove the ultimate battle between good and evil has transformed the world. Writing four days after the attack, he prays that the new order to come will be forged with mercy, mercy for those who will be its heirs, for "the wide-eyed children." That no country can escape the ravages of the current conflict, that no citizen is immune to evil, is emphasized by Dannie Abse in "Refugee." In the work, Abse defines a nation in the abstract; suffering is conveyed in images of violence. The unnamed countries, the violated victims, the despairing families—all represent nations that are unified by a common loss of peace in confronting the malevolence that would destroy them. "'In Panic as Killers Close In'" takes into account the violations and massacres committed against the guiltless worldwide. Poet Ron Charach condemns the massacre and violation of the guiltless by common thugs who justify their actions in the name of God. Jerome W. Freeman reminds us in "The Trojans" that the local conflict recorded in the glorious verses of Homer was a futile one; the universal meaning we carry with us is that the global hostilities endured by current society are no different.

Whatever it is that causes armies to clash—ideologies, territorial claims, natural resources—Laureate and Pulitzer Prize–winning poet Richard Eberhart identifies those strengths that enable us to endure. He points to poetry as being among our nation's most precious resources. He notes, "It has no energy crisis, possessing a potential that will last as long as the country. Its power is equal to that of any country in the world."[4]

Our sampling of the works included in this new anthology reveals many common topics and themes. The connections are not accidents. They result from a shared vision of experience that may be attributed to the medical gaze. We have been both amazed and delighted by our exploration of the contemporary world of poetry by physicians. We hope that our comments will move you to further explore the wealth of writing contained in these pages and to make discoveries that you will find particularly valuable for you. We hope, especially, that you will enjoy our selections.

NOTES

1. Paul Engle, "William Carlos Williams, M.D.," *Horizon* 1 (March 1959), 60–61.

2. William Osler, *Aequanimitas* (Philadelphia: P. Blakisston's Sons, 1932), 3–11.

3. C. D. Leake, *Percival's Medical Ethics* (New York: Robert E. Krieger Publishing Company, 1975), 71.

4. Richard Eberhart, quoted in http://apnews.myway.com//article/20050612/D8AM78400.html (accessed June 2005).

primary care

DANNIE ABSE

▪ AMONG A HEAP OF STONES

"I've lost my soul," the sick man said,
(the soul does not like a sick body)
"but somewhere in the world, some winter place,
surely there must be a potion, or an herb,
or a mineral, which can cure me?"

Alert, we came to a tame cold wilderness
(in every city there is so much rubble)
and I, a doctor, picked up a nameless stone,
weighed it in my hand, felt it, smelt it,

then chose another, one almost the same,
but darker, odorless, and touched by frost
—as if there were (speak to me of music)
such a thing as a stone mysterious
among a heap of stones which, if found,
would let a man reclaim what he has lost.

■ REFUGEE

What is the name of your country?
   Its frontiers keep changing.
What is the Capital of your country?
   The town where blood issued
   through the cold and hot water taps.
What is your National Anthem?
   The ancient fugue of screams.
Who are your compatriots?
   The crippled, the groping blinded,
   the wan dead not yet in their dungeons.
Who is your leader?
   Death's trumpet-tongued fool.
What is the name of your son?
   Despair.
What is the name of your daughter?
   Derangement.
Why is your husband not with you?
   He raised high the pleading
   white flag of surrender.

A DOCTOR'S REGISTER

And yet God has not said a word!
—R. Browning, "Porphyria's Lover"

Half asleep, you recalled a fading list
of girls' sweet names. Now to old women
these names belong—some whom you tumbled and kissed
in summer's twilit lanes or hidden by heather.
You were a youth who never stayed long for Gwen or for Joyce, for Rita or Ruth
and there were others too, on a lower register.

Then, suddenly, a robust, scolding voice
changed your dream's direction and the weather:
"That much morphia, doctor? Wrong, wrong."

Surprised to discover your eyes still shut
you wondered which dead patient or what
(whose accusing son and when?) as any
trusted doctor would who did not murder
any pleading one with sovereign impunity.

"I found a thing to do," said the lover
of Porphyria. *Porphyria?* Awake you add
the other pretty names too: Anuria,
Filaria, Leukemia, Melanoma,
Sarcoma, Euthanasia, amen.

ADVICE TO A FIRST-YEAR MEDICAL STUDENT

When he taught me to put in an intravenous line,
the fourth-year student advised,
think of how it will end,
work backwards: *the tape,*
                the tubing,
                the fluid flowing freely,
                the bag,
                the needle,
                the alcohol prep.
Anticipate everything you need.
Like a spell I repeated these words:
anticipate everything I need;
anticipate need
everything I;
anticipate
I
need
everything.
I dreamt
a white wall of bricks
on which I stood all night
to watch over my patients
thinking of how it would end.
I slept in my shoes.

Even now.
Insomnia rooted in visions
of the end.
So much anticipation
so much everything
so much I need.

SCANT RESOURCES

Not knowing how to comfort her
I held her wiry hand
and told her about the camphor-hunters
pushing through the hemp,
pairs of wagtails that each morning
hexed me when I gained the car.

Rescue from this old folks' home
was out of the question.
Her jaws worked, stunned beyond belief
at the same old hump of hills,
the always-on TV, a day-glo flicker
almost bigger than the window.

Some were out hunting their deaths.
Pain was something she'd dug from the Book.
It was busily being metamorphosed
into mineral seams and faults.
Who'd expect a witchetty grub totem
standing in a field of maize?

One day, we all go too deep
into ourselves, despite the counsel
of the hoary medicine-man
and our hapless mothers, beseeching us.
We go into the thick night
and then the only landscape, older than us.

The camphor-hunters were smoking out a hive.
I touched underwater tree-taps,
strips of song on the upper branches,
years ruffling the surface
of a life as it slowly lapsed into the sump,
bitter, defiant, its bed on its back.

▓ A SHINING

It was tenure in the wilderness at High Mark farm,
up-country marshes, fens, bracken, sheep stomps.

    I went there to give bad news
    and watch what they'd do with it.

Like that time the family stopped at the road's edge
and something still breathed in the wreckage.

    Silence fluttered across the room—
    a sparrow among the high rafters.

They'd already worked out the terse coded message
darkening the door of the hay-bound paddock.

    Somehow I'd trampled on their eggs
    and cut a furrow across the carpet.

I listened to my own voice, a damp dishcloth
squeezed out on whatever might have been shining.

    Better gobsmacked by hard rain, one said,
    than the horse doctor of happenstance.

HOW JFK KILLED MY FATHER

Within recent medical times psychologic investigations have reawakened interest in the psychological settings in which illness develops. Reports in the literature have singled out loss as a precipitating factor in a variety of disorders . . . including ulcerative colitis.
—Arthur H. Schmale, Jr., M.D., Psychosomatic Medicine

It was a time when men wore fedoras
banded on the crown, each band with a feather
tucked into a bow, and inside,
sweat bands carved from calf skins
with their sweet smell of animal and earth.
I remember the photo over my grandfather's desk,
a sepia toned panorama shot
from his ninth-floor factory window,
Broadway below a surge of ticker-tape
and hats tossed in the air for FDR,
hats pouring into the street, hats
waved in exaltation, hats
taking off like America.

After two war-time winters in Greenland
my father came home, hat in hand,
and bought the sweat band business,
made it grow like his young family, presidents
and hopefuls motorcading down Broadway:
Truman in a Scala wool Hamburg,
Ike's bald head steamed in fur felt,
Stevenson's ideals lost in the glory
of a two-inch-brimmed Stetson.
But when thick-haired Kennedy
rode top down and bare-headed,
men all over America took off their hats
in salute, in praise and imitation,
flung them into the street forever.
Hat factories closed quiet as prayer books,
and loss lingered in my father's guts
like unswept garbage after a big parade.

Years later, yarmulke on my head,
they asked me to view him in his coffin.
I can still see his face shaved smooth as calf skin,
his dark suit, crisp white shirt and tie,
how I laughed that they dressed him for eternity
without a hat. And I can still hear
the old men murmur in the graveyard,
Kennedy did it to him,
fedoras held close to their leathered hearts.

■ PIANO MUSIC

for Howard Kanner, M.D., 1945–1996

A flag at half-mast, tissues piled
in the OR lounge, the hallway gasps:
What were his risk factors?
No one dared say it out loud,
how we tallied our own frailties,
clear for an instant,
like skywriting before a wind.

On the day he could not know
would be his last, he traced healing scars
with eye and fingertip, cut new wounds
with clean hands, alive
with the snap of latex gloves,
the precise steel scalpel and rongeur.
Between cases, he confided in me:
a wish to learn piano, an instrument
where the choices are black and white.
And he laughed as he ate a peach,
the sugary juice glistening
on his hand, his tongue
tasting each scrubbed finger.
I don't know who he touched
between the pleasures of a peach
and the call to 9-1-1,
what music he heard as he waited.

9

1898

From a ton of pitchblende
dumped at the edge of pine-woods,
Marie Curie fills her vats
and begins a four year stirring.
She boils hot miasma
down to thimbles of crystal radium
until the lab fills with the glow of decay.
At night, avoiding the moon's spell,
Marie and Pierre bathe
in flickering blue silhouettes
that glow in their tubes *like faint fairy lights.*
I can see them kiss like lovers before a fire,
passions aflame, her marrow burning to scar.

1917

Huddled in Belgian trenches
where time has stopped,
soldiers count the numbers
radiating from their watches,
deadly as mustard gas,
comforting as any light in darkness.
Back home, their sweethearts
long for safe returns, yearn
for glow-in-the-dark light pulls.

1918

50 girls hunch at wooden desks
in the Radium Dial Company, Ottawa, Illinois,
hair cut short, heads aligned like an army in review,
not a soldier older than 20,
wooden trays beside them filled with clocks
arranged like cupcakes waiting to be iced.
They mix paint from powdered base,
lip-point brushes with long licks

into tips fine enough to paint time,
two hundred fifty dials a day,
five and a half days each week,
a penny and a half per dial.
Covered with a thin powder
that *puts a glow in your cheeks*,
they paint their buttons, fingernails, teeth.
Beneath the stardust, boys gravitate
to their radiant blue bodies.

1925

Confused bones bond Radium tight,
and it singes their core
until jaws break, teeth rot,
wounds grow purulent without healing.
The company claims safety.
Dentists lie through their teeth.
And one hundred Radium Girls are dead.

1938

A woman is stretched out on her sick bed.
Five former workers encircle her,
arms folded, looking down at the figure
whose eyes are closed and could pass for dead.
A dark-suited man sits and stares
directly at her closed eyes but doesn't touch her.
One woman holds a comma of white hand
while the others stand inert.
On the wall behind the group
hangs a cheap picture of a pine forest
my eyes search for a pile of pitchblende.

1998

Motherless since six, a 70-year-old daughter
walks her 5 A.M. mile to the Ottawa cemetery
and tends the grass on her mother's grave.
Argonne National Laboratory dug here last month.
Six feet down, bones still tick
in the earth's dark pocket.

BLOOD SONG

I keep asking
and no one seems to know:
    Why do they keep coming
    to get their hearts?

Down here in the Surgical Pathology Lab
we don't see patients often.
The walls here quiver with anticipation
when one is coming   like the stunned walls
of their heart came quivering in a stainless pan
the week before.
We simply don't know what to say.
Would they like it in a jar?
a brown paper bag?   wet or dry?
formalin or alcohol?

Years ago they came for their gallstones
to set them out   split and multifaceted
    strictly ornamental
But a heart?   flabby and failed
without its thumping gallop
on the coffee table?

One woman, just out of Recovery
anorexia hanging loosely on her
wanted only to hold her old heart.
"My diary wouldn't be complete without a look,"
she said as she turned it under the fluorescent light
pale and forlorn like fatigued metal
its concrete arteries   dark worms on the surface.
She spoke so softly of how   long ago
it had rhythmically pounded
over the wet springtime pastures of her youth.

Some come to bury them
but most—like her—come to look

pay their respects   then
turning toward the door
they leave with another heart
their long-awaited harvest
singing its new blood song.

ENTITLEMENTS

Middle age comes upon us unaware,
The years begin to slide by unannounced,
The extra breath it takes to climb the stair,

The lost or misplaced key, the graying hair,
The familiar phrase blocked or mispronounced.
Middle age comes upon us unaware.

Like tax returns we need time to prepare,
Life-long pleasures take time to be renounced.
The extra breath it takes to climb the stair,

The modest paunch, the cautionary air,
All apply in reckoning our accounts;
Middle age comes upon us unaware,

We need to take out time to get us there,
We need to deal in debits and amounts,
The extra breath it takes to climb the stair.

We need a moment, coming up for air,
To pause, to measure, even to denounce
(Middle age comes upon us unaware)
The extra breath it takes to climb the stair.

PLAGUE DOCTOR

The habit of despair is worse than despair itself.
—Camus

Why had he chosen to stay,
Worn the mantle of Physician
In the midst of pestilence,

When all the others had gone?
Not for any love of humanity.
He knew too much

Of degradation and deceit.
Did he need a reason beyond his calling?
He thought of Pericles in plague time.

Pulling long leather gloves above his elbows,
He donned the broad-brimmed hat,
Placed the beaked leather mask upon his face.

Smell of myrrh from its carapace filled his nostrils,
Shrouding fumes exuded by pyres of the dead.
Gazing through thick lenses of the mask,

Insulated from contagion in his robes,
Percussion wand in hand,
He ventured out amongst the dying.

▪ NURSING HOME

Here the walls are thin
as birthdays.
There are no distinctions.

Handsome soldiers fade
in frames of the same war.
Cards repeat each other's verses
in the same drawer.

When you look
everyone withdraws
like yesterday
like the light beneath the door.

Little comfort you are their nightmare
long before they are yours.

RADIOLOGY

Butterflies.
Before going out on stage
Before getting married
Before giving grand rounds
Before opening up the envelope on Match Day
Before my son's brain scan is read.

A 7 year old schoolboy.
That's how she described him in her note.
Fortunately, intellect is superb.

"Bony structures are prominent all around, consistent with strong-
headedness.
There is a well-defined locus of art projects, exceeding the upper limit of
normal in size.
Prominent also is the hand-holding nucleus, which usually has involuted
almost completely by this age.
Both hemispheres are equal in size, but appear hypertrophied, suggesting
persistent competition with each other. This is typically found in
unusually gifted children, or in boys with a female sibling. Clinical
correlation suggested.
Strong signal intensity is noted in the region of hand-eye coordination,
typical for conditions such as Game Boy Syndrome.
Background structures show an unusually dense collection of giggle cells
and rests of kindness."

At times like this I retreat to that primitive life raft I was raised on: please
God (whoever and whatever you are, if I am asking something this
important, you deserve the upper case), please help us all through this.
Please don't let this be something horrible. I don't want that for him. He
deserves more. My girl doesn't deserve to be a sole survivor. Whatever it is
will be hard enough to handle.

Doctor, just show me the giggle cells.
I want
to see
the giggle cells.

WHAT I WOULD GIVE

What I would like to give them for a change
is not the usual prescription with
its hubris of the power to restore,
to cure; what I would like to give them, ill
from not enough of laying in the sun
not caring what the onlookers might think
while feeding some banana to their dogs
what I would like to offer them is this,
not reassurance that their lungs sound fine,
or that the mole they've noticed change is not
a melanoma, but instead of fear
transfigured by some doctorly advice
I'd like to give them my astonishment
at sudden rainfall like the whole world weeping,
and how ridiculously gently it
slicked down my hair; I'd like to give them that,
the joy I felt while staring in your eyes
as you learned epidemiology
(the science of disease in populations),
the night around our bed like timelessness,
like comfort, like what I would give to them.

QUESTIONS FOR THE WEATHER

in memory of the victims of the terrorist attacks
of 11 September 2001

To the wind: remember us. Who's not to say
the airplane roaring overhead in fact is
Armageddon? The wind is cool today,
a kind of calm before the last attack.
The wind is hurling birds across the sky,
enacting distance, pretending what can fly
is always beautiful. Who's not to say
that what we can remember when we die
is really just a single moment? Not a life
of great accomplishments, but a cool wind
that touched us once, less urgently than love,
but as familiar as a long-lost friend.
The wind does not remember us. Yet we'll
remember it, distantly, desperately.

THE CARDIAC EXAM

Before the brainless heart gives out,
I realized while listening
To hers—I guess I understood
Its plaintive language passably,

Unlike the Spanish from her mouth,
That drowning, soft, unloosened song
It wants to do some lasting good,
It wants never again to bleed,

It wants to float up just outside
The lonesome body that contains it.
To swell with joyful empathy,
Re-tell the cancer's seeding of

Her pericardium—a wide
Expanse of sweetest Cuban fruit
That feeds starved throngs, not emptiness
Unfilled by muffled beats of love

So distant I begin to hear
The music of a dying few,
Of how not one of us survived
Their murders, bodies choking swamps.

The germ of knowledge is in here:
Her failing organ is in you
Just as in me, her blue-green eyes
One world, a promise to be kept.

ROBERT CARROLL

SHOW AND TELL

So much depends upon
the red baby
tumbling—
my father,
my son.
And me—
tumbling in space,
tumbling in time.
That's what it's like
to have a kid.

I know a child who's dying,
not in his body,
but in his mind.
He's dying,
scared he's dying,
his mouth a potato.
He was smart once,
he knows, he sees.
The trees appall him now.

His father watches in horror
as he takes pills from jars,
his eyes big as knotholes.

We all live up close.
We all make history.
No one's out of the loop.
No one.

HAL

How many are there like you,
awkward six-four mantis frame,
bobbing head high above the crowds, or folded
high-kneed on a seat in an endless subway,
a last worn volume of Dostoevsky to your name?
You changed appearance with each mood,
a series of brilliant heads:
some hairy, some shaved,
each anguished, and off the mark.

Your inventions!
A straw hooked up to a vacuum cleaner
pulled snot faster than a head-cold replaced it.
And your performance art:
a slide-show of wrinkled blank pages, magnifications
of things no one would think to show,
set to music.

Your suicide, however long predicted, was sudden,
like the white-water rafting
you tried once on a lark,
complete strangers howling across you
as you offered your finely shaped skull
and proud tartar cheekbones
to cool passages
marked by rocks.

▓ "IN PANIC AS KILLERS CLOSE IN"

I write this tonight because for the past six weeks,
using scalpel blade and alcohol,
moleskin and Scotch tape,
I have been shaving at the base
of my son's plantar warts,
a wincing act of care
that skirts the base of cruelty

and because, in this morning's *Star*,
of a photo titled LOST HOPE.
Sleepless haunted eyes
festooned by windblown hair,
Algerian Assia Bayeesh looks out at the reader,
holding a tiny girl who pulls at her sleeve, revealing
a stretch of lacy cotton.
"Assia Bayeesh, 18, clutches a girl
pulled from a terrorist's fire in Sidi Rais.
The cousin who saved the girl was killed for the act."

Who is taking young women as sex slaves
in *zawaj al mutaa*, "Marriages of pleasure"
that strip the jewels from their victims?

Who is hurling babies from rooftops
into makeshift bonfires
while chanting "God is great!"
—*Mujahideen?*

Who is slitting villagers' throats
or, as they themselves ask,
Qui *tué* qui?

The Armed Islamic Group?
The army? Local thugs
the army uses
to justify its presence?

They know too well who it is.

Nor are we all innocence.
As teens, my friends and I had our "cruelty index"
that licensed jokes at the expense of the infirm
(careful never to be overheard)
disregarding how our own people
wandered the Earth in black
receiving a gypsy's welcome.

I write this tonight to forgo
my people's monopoly on holocaust,
to say that again and again the world stares up
at the mustachioed leering face of massacre:
Germany, Russia, Poland,
Armenia, Cambodia, Rwanda,
Iraq versus Iran, with keys to heaven issued
to the first wave of teenagers to rush the enemy tanks;
the take-no-prisoners Nintendo wars of Uncle Sam.
Tonight it burns in some far-off desert land
that expat Canadians have fled
to sleep, well-covered
in their home-country's beds.

Tonight I want my country
to let in no fanatics, torturers, female circumcisers,
acid-in-a-young-girl's-face avengers,
no one who despises with "us against them,"
I want a moral means test, *a border!*
a place for any who passively resist
the call to tempered steel,
for those who do not know where to begin
to defend themselves or their sleeping kin.
Lovely Assia Bayeesh and little cousin,
enter as refugees.
May we stop your deep-brown eyes from staring
and staring at it again.

▨ THE OLD CARDIOLOGY DREAM

Last night I had
the old cardiology dream,
a baby born with six hearts.
So many valves that could falter!
And how rare,
the necessary synchrony.

Baby, I will cherish you,
one-man percussion band that you are,
and devote my life
to seeing yours through.
May none of your frail pink hearts
break mine.

FIVE TASKS

for my brother

1. Say Good-Bye

You called me at work to ask for a loan
And said good-bye as sweetly as if I'd said yes.
I was unhappy, & probably rude.
It was the last time we talked.

2. Express Forgiveness

I forgive you for stepping over the edge,
Wearing a roofer's safety harness
Clipped stylishly to nothing,
Momentary angel over Arizona.

When you were seven
You flew the swingset outside
Our Chilean house through an earthquake
As walls and ceilings collapsed into themselves.
"More, make it do that again!"

Your life was not as short as I feared
Nor as long as I hoped.

3. Request Forgiveness

Forgive me for not lending you the money
To buy that motorcycle,
For not admiring your poetry,
For never taking a photograph of you with my sons.
Forgive me for not wrestling with you into more
Sunsets the summer before I was drafted.
Forgive me for being your imitation angel,
For leaving you with the elephant in the living room.
Forgive me for living.

4. Affirm Affection

I love you
For being obvious about loving me
When I was fifteen and
Thought I couldn't bear to be loved.
You were too young to know better.

You were so alive,
Your death seemed impossible—
If you could die everyone would.

5. Express Gratitude

Thank you for giving me back
My lost family and Montana,
Where we scattered your ashes
According to your instructions:
Up Big Creek Canyon and
On the hundred-year
Flood plain of the Bitterroot River.

West Yellowstone burned all the week
Of your death, frosting windshields white in July.
Now, when I visit—and I visit often—
I do work I love,
While I stay in a lodge built ten years ago
Of first-growth timber
Salvaged from that fire.

Now I see: living is a kind of slow burning,
And love is what we salvage from the fire.

ACUTE MYOCARDIAL INFARCTION

The electrical activity of the heart
of a man who was alive yesterday
is legible to me now,
written on graph paper
in a language it has
taken me ten years to learn.

A spear pierced the left side
of his last good dream
and he never truly woke.

DO NO HARM

A spider in the sink is stunned. The light.
My size. Big sucker, brown. The body
bulges. Otherwise, it's squat. If I wait
a few minutes without moving, it'll glide
over the dry porcelain, attending
to its needs. Why do these spiders appear?
This one must have dropped from the ceiling
on a sticky thread. It couldn't have been
exploring. Spiders don't, unless . . . looking
for water? Attracted to a new spot?
I don't think so. Out in the open sink,
vulnerable at any moment
to flood, this arachnid is as good as dead.
What kind of being? There is no way
to understand how it feels. It may eat
its own eggs. It hasn't friends. The sheen
of the porcelain means nothing to it.
Act without thought. I will turn the tap
to the right temperature and pull out
my razor. I could switch off the light and wait
for the spider to leave, or flick it up
with a Kleenex. But I don't. I let
the torrent loose and turn for a moment
to the shower, so I can't see the spider
struggling and sliding, as its whole life,
for all I know, flashes in front of it.

■ THAT INTERN DREAM

I had the intern dream again last night,
restored to white, but decades older
than that group of docs I hadn't met.

Halfway through, it seemed I kept
clutching a fear so tight, my smile was tin.
Nor had I seen a single patient yet.

At midnight rumpled interns ate
cold spaghetti, bread, and juice. From a seat
across the room, I scanned their faces,

convinced they didn't know my hideous sin.
In fact, I had never learned to put
a tube in place, or make an incision.

Instead I read a book. Emergency!
My name was called. A code. I had to run,
but which direction? The route I took

was wrong, and I reversed. My pants collapsed.
My coat and shirt were gone. I jockeyed
to the corridor in underpants and socks.

What chance I had of saving face was lost.
The call was cardiac. My father lay
gasping for his breath, but I'd never seen

a Swan put in, or learned resuscitation.
Emptiness arose. I ran away.
Lilies choked the room. I slept. I woke.

■ PHRENOLOGY

Concavities and lumps above my ear
speak narratives I never would have known
before relentless loss of all my hair

turned truth about my scalp so baldly clear—
the story of my life is in the bone.
Convexities and slumps above my ear

identify the site of passion: here.
Like tenacity and hope, it's in a zone
invisible before the loss of hair

writ large the heady script of character.
Depression, fancy, awkwardness intone
complexity that's bunched above my ear

for you to read. Your gentle fingers, dear,
interpret my desire and mine alone.
My scalp is blessed to have no trace of hair.

It shines with gratitude—I love your care
for this old scalp, though never have I won
a way to read the bumps above *your* ear,
which even now are swathed in silver hair.

▪ FOUR PERFECT QUARTERS

when I lost the green ash twelve
summers ago you came into the yard
with a saw and a deal—
for half the haul you'd
cut it all into ready rounds
and teach me to maul split, to
aim for the inviting cleft
let tool and gravity do the work
breathe, bend knees, relish

the way the four quarters fall apart, the look
and smell of startled heartwood
the flat dull ring of a thrown log on its
partners, like tumbling children's blocks
a siren song that always called you back
to my yard or kept you in yours
working other hauls from other deals

I don't remember when I stopped
hearing your hammer or smelling
your November smoke or knew about the
six heme grams, ten sigmoid inches
forty-seven pounds you lost, and
thousands of portal triads sliced
microtome thin, or how long since the
stiff-suited day I walked yard to yard past
your pile—a blue tarp capped peak above
border tangle of honeysuckle and wild rose
—to sit inside a circle of cakes with dew
beads slipping off polished shoes and tell
stories stacked tall enough to last many winters

but wish you could have seen me with
my own saw after the May storm took
the black walnut by the fence, or been lured
today by the claves clack under a July cicada
sun to watch me work the few rounds I bid

from millers and carvers, or sweat with
me over that stuck-wedge stubborn

or been home to see the four perfect
quarters I laid next to your dwindle of
parched gray oak, to admire the way the cut
bared the grain, pointing like a candle flame, like
church steeple, the light brown almost
yellow, the dark almost violet, you would have
warned me to keep on my gloves, that the wet
bark would stain my hands

■ TRISOMY 13

What is time to you? Correct
my genes; rearrange base pairs
of my base and acid into normal life

for your dear absence's sake: someone,
no one, make the wheel of my misfortune
(which chance misspun in sperm or egg)

spin again: unloving God, let me live;
change the straw of my affliction into
nuggets of pure gold; Rumpelstiltskin

(you have been called worse) let me live!
Take the curse, remove the extra ware
that wrenches this computer, prevents

flesh to be even a desperate "me"—
for I am a monster. I have no hope.
They look through the window and see

a thing with a cleft lip; they disappear.
My brain's faulty wires beat faith; poor
protoplasm doctors call me; "Have another kid!"

How could you do this and still be wise and good?
It's not your fault, I know, you don't exist—
And they'll go on, relearn trust and love

again. And me? Sometimes chance seems savager
than Nazi doctors. Choosing life nevertheless,
they come back, half-smiling now; have you?

■ ON A WIZARDLESS WARD

About a billion viruses and one
scared diploid version of God's image
struggle under covers. Vast Ocean,

I am too young, says a drop of free will
cascading into automaton. Swell;
come, says the encroaching jungle, swell

despite Lasix and drown. Who's that?
The woman who's known me for thirty-three years
stares at my bed like a stranger—

All dying people are frogs.
Here he comes, says the other blank side of the wall—
I can't stay like this. And you won't,

says Death; the Good Witch of the North's
wand in an ancient, chthonic hand
waves over his head and transforms him—

Another semiconscious traveler
halfway to Oz on a bedpan
falls back to Kansas; then Kansas dissolves.

■ ANATOMY

*after hearing a poem that compared women
to deep underground mines*

Women are not holes
nor caverns nor mouths
no part of us is hollow

when your mouth is closed
it is not hollow
your tongue fills it entirely

the womb is a pear-shaped muscle
the space inside it is a flat space
like the space inside an envelope

a term baby fills it entirely
tightly packed, it can barely move

when the child's feet leave
within those same seconds
the muscular wall contracts down

when the placenta leaves
the uterus is a solid ball
the size of a coconut
and everyday thereafter
shrinks by two fingerbreadths
until it is again
a pear-sized muscle
with a flat space inside it

the vulva is a flat bowl
part the lips and you see
no cave nor hollow
but
a flattened living envelope

the vagina is a short flat tube
about three inches long
whose walls touch

of course it can expand
and take on the shape
of whatever is allowed into it
from above or below

but when we are walking about
or sleeping or sitting
or talking over coffee or thinking
women are not holes.

■ ITCH

e lascia pur grattar dov'e la rogna.
(and let them scratch wherever they itch.)
—Dante, Paradiso, Canto XVII, line 129

Itch is pain's bratty kid brother
with squirt-gun and feather
to splash or tickle the backs
of respectable necks when we're
not looking. It grabs the wire
reserved for disasters
and gabs on it for hours.
Pain has dignity—
the martyr's groans are holy;
we comfort the wounded
but an itch? We laugh
at the twisting, reaching
for the remote spot, above all,
the scratching.
In Dante's Paradise one can rub
a prickling patch at will,
but in earthly hell
our pretense is always
interrupted: a nettle
drawn at random
across pristine skin demands
to be scraped, starts again
as the fingernail moves off.
That's why we name
our chief devil Old Scratch.

ANOTHER DRIVE-BY

Drive-by birth. This mother snares a cab,
Shoots up, delivers, leaves her baggage
Backseat to the world. Boy born. Tab
Unpaid. The driver hasn't disengaged
The gears. Paramedics cut the cord.
The taxi twitches, swears, then disappears.
Sirens swaddle them and us in sordid
City night. Small body in arrears
For drugs. Drugs lace a smile across a face
Devoid of motherhood, numb to need.
She nearly rolls onto him, takes his place.
We take her in to detox, warm, to feed
A son. Withdrawal fuels a newborn thirst.
Milky, dawn suckles day by dying first.

CARRYING ON

In an off-handed fashion
he sometimes reports
suffering joint pains during
the eighty-eighth year
of getting things done.

When I casually suggest
a trial of some aspirin,
he answers
that lots of folks
use that stuff
as a stick of some kind,
but he never thought
much of it.

He's gnarled and weathered
making his way through
life and pain with the easy
certainty of someone
on the threshold of heading
somewhere else.

▩ THE TROJANS

It's a hard thing to suffer a war
for a woman we neither know
nor love. We were proud when
Paris bested the dirty Greeks
with her abduction, but that was
before this siege and paltry rations.

Our gods and old Priam tell us
the portents are promising.
But we are fatigued, yearning
to leave these walls and walk
along the beach alone.

Yesterday Helen passed by
the rampart looking bored and
beautiful in the morning sun.
Crazy Cassandra followed
apace calling out jealousy
and doom. Our attentions
were distracted.

Now we hear the enemy's
strange calls, amid pounding
clamor on the plains. This
latest project will surely fail
like their earlier machinations.
Maybe then the horde will return
vanquished to their distant home
and deserted women, if they will
take them back again.

BENIGN FASICULATIONS

One day, unprovoked,
  a small snake ripples
in my thigh, unbidden as a tic
  around the eye. Something
broken to congeal the honey
  in my flesh,
a beehive gone awry.

Under a harsh light, you
  report the nexus spread
like a brush-fire's nascent flame
  to calves and head.
A syncopated wave
  of muscular babble
unrecruited by anything
  I've done or said, and then
I tell you I'm dead;
  a droplet poised
at the end of life's spout.
  Just a few months
'til my spinal cord rots,
  breath is snuffed, and crawlers
pick my femurs clean.

At night I shout,
  pursued by visions
of catacombs, of men I've tended,
  slowly wasted to the bone,
wide-eyed as inmates
  from the camps,
begging God to take them home.

What injustice
  this chooses me,
must be what Lou Gehrig thought
  and I think now
in my psychotic bloom.

You, merciful queen
  hold my head in the unraveling
of this delicate thread;
  my tears repentant
for the births and sunsets not seen,
  arrivals and migrations,
aspirations left unsaid.

I fall asleep on a spread of nails,
  pierced by every tip-toe
of this animal beneath my skin.
  Until salvation comes
from a colleague's keen mind
  and calm hand. Who declares
this invasion, benign.

EPITHALAMIUM

The first time I ever saw a brain
all pink and throbbing in its ivory safe,
bulged through a hole the neurosurgeon made
to let the pressure out and so to save
my aunt who hit her head against a wall.
I was transfixed by curiosity;
that holy ordering of ridge and rut
fed by more tributaries than the sea,
repository for her every thought.

Hoping to find a grail of the mind,
I've searched the cryptic swirls that brain-waves sign,
watched nerve cells sprout like tadpoles through a scope,
and patients seized by toxins, tics and strokes.
The nature of a thought remains unknown;
what leap occurs between the ear and tongue,
elusive as chimera or a bowl
of sky that fills me to the brim, the brain
must be the mortal bridegroom of the soul.

◼ SUICIDE ON CHRISTMAS EVE

After the doctor, the steam-cleaners,
more usefully. I drive home to bed
through intersections sequined with glass:
it's Christmas Eve, season of donor organs.

What is the meaning of life? I shake you
gently awake. What answer would satisfy?
You mumble, yawning, from Your Side.
To understand is to be bored, you say,
practicing, perhaps, for Speech Night.
Knowledge is a kind of exhaustion, you say.

A child enters our room: is it morning yet?
Not Yet. In another room the lights of the Tree
wink colorfully, and when the telephone rings
again, it is almost, but not quite, in time.

■ ODE TO ALCOHOL

You are the eighth
and shallowest
of the seven seas,
a shriveled fragmented ocean
dispersed into bottles, kegs, casks,
warm puddles in lanes behind pubs:
a chain of ponds.
Also a kind of spa,
a very hot spring:
medicinal waters to be taken
before meals, with meals, after meals,
without meals;
chief cure for gout,
dropsy, phlegm, bad
humors, apoplexy, rheumatism
and chief cause of all the same.
At best you make lovely mischief:
wetter of cunts,
deflater of cocks.
At worst you never know when to stop:
wife-beater, mugger of innocents,
chief mitigating circumstance
for half the evil in the world.
All of which I know too well
but choose to ignore,
remembering each night only this advice:
never eat on an empty stomach;
for always you make me a child again
sentimental, boring
and for one happy hour very happy
sniffing out my true character like a dog:
my Sea of Tranquility,
always exactly shallow enough to drown in.

■ HEALTH CARE

When Jake bleeds into his lungs I realize
(though I've known him and his mother and
his brain tumor and his chemo and his veins
too long) I don't know them well enough
to ask: *How hard d'you want us to try here?*

Four A.M. and Jake's refusing O_2, let alone
the ET tube. His BP's as high as his
blood count is low. He's spluttering: *Let me
f . . . ing die! And I'm not your f . . . ing sweetheart!*
Yelling at me between bloody coughs.

Too right, you're not. So how come I'm using
such language of endearment with this
thirteen-year-old monster who, from the look
of him and his mother, never knew what it was
to be held, let alone hugged, in his life.

The room's choked with people, machines, clutter,
the floor awash: used and dropped syringes,
leaking plastic saline bags, blood from his lungs,
veins, arteries, paper (penciled records of orders
bellowed, lab readings, torn-off EKG strips).

His mother won't leave his left side,
curses us, and him, with a stream of
f . . . ing a . . . h . . . s. While we struggle, sliding and
slipping, to get mask in place, arms strapped,
four of us to hold down the flailing feet.

Meanwhile, back in the nurses' changing room
(unlocked at this hour: we pinned down
the time later), someone else is at work:
lifting credit cards, a checkbook, fifty dollars
from a student's wallet: a good haul.

▪ LAST RITES

Sunday morning: in the drive-through
outside the Emergency Room idle
four red and white county ambulances
that double as fire trucks, engines puttering
their impromptu four-part harmony.

Mr. Mackie, erstwhile Hurricanes linebacker,
squats in the ER doorway, hiding from the heat,
scrunches the frail plastic bag that holds
his three-year-old daughter's underwear,
embroidered with Peter Rabbit motifs.

Soon he'll head home, lift them from their bag,
stand over his sink, wash the blood from them.
The ambulance driver joins his mate; they start
to sluice down the flooring with their hoses.
After the vomit and blood the water runs clear.

AUS-LAN

Australian sign language

My deaf friend said to me: our conversations
    are all overheard, everywhere we speak.
He teaches me the sign for Sydney: the shape

of a harbor bridge, skin webbing blue water.
    I hear a quiet voice in my hands
in the silence when I am speaking

and foam, rubber, snow, and glycerin
    seem softer in the fingering span
than spoken words falling short of what they name.

I once saw a baby catching sunlight in his hands—
    everywhere the child touched
he laughed at what he could not touch

until language wheeled his pram away
    and he learned that silhouettes and sun
were called *chair* and *where.*

Precisely, in mother tongue, we categorize
    the conch shells, sea hollows
the safety pins and taboos.

My friend said: I will teach you
    what you need to know . . .
other signs belong only to the deaf.

He teaches me the sign Forget
    it is a fist placed against the right temple
the hand opening, flicking sun away from the head.

CAMBODIANS CELEBRATE THE BUDDHIST
NEW YEAR ONCE AGAIN

After incense drapes a smoky praise on the buddhas,
after food is brought on silver trays to priests,
after children ride the tame elephant and old men—
those few who survived—gamble at tiles,

the promenade begins.

Hundreds of people on motorbikes
hum along the Mekong riverside,
pass Wat Thom on Phnom Penh's solitary hill,
amble the French boulevards whose flame trees
ignite each spring, then circle
the goat-and-mango pagoda, and return to the river . . .

over and over until it spells night.

Whole families glide on single bikes; their children
clasped together like still-warm slices of bread.
Young women—side-saddle, coal-black hair loose
to the waist or pinned by chrysanthemums—
barely touch the thighs and shoulders of young men.

I wish I could remember the High Holy Days,

when daughters of Jerusalem danced barefoot
in groves of figs, arbors of grapes, lilies in their hair,
in linen robes spinning up at their ankles,
singing out to the young men of Nazareth,
of Bethlehem. They danced after the sheep
was slaughtered, burnt whole and offered: a sacrifice

the Bible names The Holocaust, "all consumed."

TUSCAN STILL LIFE, WITH SHEEP

If the dog turns up we'll watch it snooze—
content to let the sheep bells jubilate
from pasture to pasture.
He'll come too, in his crumpled Peugeot,
cupping a smoke in the morning cold.

Down by the homeward lea where the sheep swill
water from claw-foot tubs filled from a nearby spring,
he's built a splendid grotto—chicken wire
dressed in morning glory—protecting
tomatoes, rucola, sage.

Sinking into a punched-out couch, he croons
to his flock: "ooloo ya, ooloo ya"—
and munches on the ripe, pliant fruit
whose seedy gush dribbles over his lips.
When I begin to nibble at memories,

I hope you'll put me out in a sunny square—
my cap, my cane, my pillowed chair—
where I can make sheep's eyes at *ragazze*
walking saucy, tossing their hair.   Love without desire:
Will it ever come? Will it *ever* come?

■ EXPUNGE

Never having suckled a child, she thought breasts were a waste of time to begin with. After the mastectomy, she refused to remember what his love letters said, or where they were hidden. Her chest prepped for radiation, she wondered what to do about those purple-red marks at the pool. Tamoxifen to block her estrogen, gesso to paint over her old canvases.

ELIDE

Pink field of skin, Elysian, the baby's bottom, ripe apricots, faint fur. Leave off the diaper. Elision. The tongue's slip, writing its own mind, collision of intent with the unmeant. The Asian dermatologist removes a lesion. A few snips, ellipsis, a few sutures. Dysplasia begins at home, then it wanders, elusive cells. Your old dinghy, curled scales of beige paint, swings alee. Shun the high tides, the wild eddies, tack back into the shallow cove where eluvial shore eclipses peach sunset, that glow.

■ WHAT IF LASHIKA?

Imagine this.
What if Lashika
just dropped
the role that
she's been playing
like a
coat?

What if she stopped
being the troubling
wildly borderline
seventeen-year-old
black female
she played so well
at our last meeting?

I mean imagine
her approaching me
with a big smile
like anybody else
and saying, Doctor Joy!
It's good to see you.
How you been?

And by the way,
thank you so much
for being such a help to me
at that last meeting.
It was hard
for me then.
Things are better now.

I can imagine
this. But she can't
stop being herself
as if she were
an actress instead

of an adolescent
on probation.

What I know is
(and here's the
scientific part)
neither one of us
will live long enough
for any of this
to come true.

Imagine this though.
What if an actress
were playing Lashika?
Then it might
happen for sure.

■ BLUES FOR ME

The best that can be said
is that it isn't any worse.

All these mistakes I've made
are as unintentional as yours.

Perhaps it's like he said, our son,
another one of our innocent victims.

He said he thinks an evil devil
has caused all of this to happen.

In fact, if there's an evil devil, it's
the one who keeps yelling, "Abandon ship!"

▪ BELLEVUE HOSPITAL BLUES

East River runs past Bellevue
From Spanish Harlem to the sea
Carries heavy freight and fuel oil
Runs from Harlem to the sea
And when I see those proud ships passing
I wish that river carried me

I went down to Bellevue's cellar
Water running over the stones
I pushed aside old cobwebs
And I walked on wet old stones
Saw a hundred empty cradles
Thought I heard a hundred little moans

Suicides by drowning
Where the East River runs
Suicides in winter
Where the freezing river runs
Spring will melt your prison
You'll rise like water lilies to the sun

I'll ride you easy, River
If you hold me in your hands
Ride you easy while you rock me
Easy in your hands
Cause men that ride you easy
Wake up in a strange enchanted land

The passion of the flowers
Is to kiss the lips of rain
The passion of the hours
It's just to fill my life with pain
Sweet lips of marijuana
Please ease my troubled brain

■ TRUE HISTORY OF ORPHEUS

for Vietnam, Rwanda, Yugoslavia

Once, undetected, I flowed in a crowd
across the borders of nation states.
With drought and plague and deportation
I ate my small portion.

I am that only survivor you read in the News,
widowed and orphaned in a photograph
next to the rubble.

Before that, I crisscrossed the river of the dead—
Mekong, Congo, Drina—the river of the dead
in a flak jacket, taking heavy casualties.

Back in the world again,
I enlisted in the real war
between machines and feelings.

Earliest of all, in a time before birth,
it seemed I played with consummate skill
on instruments still uninvented.
Then I fell from grace.
All the stars went out for me but one sun
that shone on my morning cradle,
my morning kiss.
My one remaining charm then:
to break and reform,
break and reform
with the surges of ocean on black rocks.

MICHAEL LIEBERMAN

PLEDGE

This is the last time I'm going to obsess about loss.
This is the last time I'm going to think about Jews dragged from
    Amsterdam, Salonika, Bucharest, Vilna, Riga, Prague, Vienna,
    Budapest, Berlin, Vichy France, Warsaw, Zagreb.
This is the last time I'm going to think about the exile of Nelly Sachs in Sweden.
This is the last time I'm going to remember the death of Paul Antschel
    and the suicide of Paul Célan.
This is the last time I'm going to think about Primo Levi.
This is the last time I'm going to imagine Bruno Schultz murdered by the Nazis.
This is the last time I'm going to reconstruct the lives of Jewish pharmacists
    and accountants, tailors, mathematicians, dressmakers, shopkeepers,
    housewives, professors, doctors, lawyers, poets, musicians,
    intellectuals, peddlers, traders, rag pickers, butchers, artisans,
    chemists, painters, and merchants during the Third Reich.
This is the last time I'm going to obsess about the deaths of Jewish children.
This is the last time I'm going to try to figure out what moves people to evil.
This is the last time I'm going to think about how fucking lucky I am and
    how many other Michael Liebermans were gassed or shot or
    strangled or bludgeoned.
This is the last time I'm going to imagine that winter predicts spring, that
    symbols of innocence mean innocence exists, that the fall can be
    splendid and prelude to a winter of quiet regeneration.
This is the last time I'm going to obsess about the beauty of flowers or
    honeydew or love or my children or family or loss.
This is the last time I'm going to think about grace and decency.
This is the last time I'm going to think about the Holocaust until
    tomorrow morning when I get up at four to read and do whatever
    it is that I am doing.

■ TIME TO DEPART

With ice storms the issue is time.
Often in Houston or St. Louis
the ice comes as rain, so that
over hours, there is an accretion,
of weight, lamination after lamination
as the water freezes on the branches,
glistening even on nights
when the moon is down.
The gradual accumulation of scale
on the limbs until their tensile strength
gives way, molecules of wood fatigue,
and the branches sagging a little
and a little more, then more,
and gaining momentum lurching
toward the ground and snapping.
This is how death blossoms
on trees during storms like these.
This is how the physics of water   ·
and mechanical force provide
time to prepare, to mourn, to depart.
Grace is a long good-bye,
a final look at the lasting beauty of the world.

▨ MONOPOLY

We set the board
on the folding table
and divide up the play money,
wrinkled from overuse.
All around the house
the sound of rain
seeps in the walls
and spatters the windows,
left open a crack
to let in the damp,
gray-green world.
My cousin Rita, thirteen,
always wins.
She chooses
the silver roadster for herself,
the iron for me,
and sets them on Go.
Fifteen years from now
she and her infant son
will glide off a slick,
Nevada highway
and disappear forever
into a gorge.
She lays the stack
of orange cards
on Chance.
I raise the dice
in my cupped hands
and rattle the air.
You have to buy
everything you land on, she says.
Everything.
It's only play money.
I throw the dice,
advance to Reading Railroad
and count out two hundred dollars.

■ HOME VISIT

I hurry to my car,
leaving behind
the noise of the hospital.
I veer around the corner,
into the small lane
and rush up the steps,
late.

I pause at the door,
hand poised at the bell as
through the window
I see him asleep
on the window bench
covered by
a carefully pieced
hand-knit blue afghan.
His wife sits
on a chair nearby
bent over,
her head on a pillow
next to his,
their white hair mingling
as they sleep.

I hesitate outside,
noticing the thick
sweet smell of
hot summer roses
hanging in the air.
I am reluctant
to disturb their
peaceful reunion.

TED MCMAHON

■ SILVER FORK, AMERICAN RIVER

In Navajo culture, each time a story is told its source is acknowledged and honored. My friend, Sue Bennett, shared with me this story of the loss of her friend Dugald Bremner.

They implore me not to go, they say
I could not bear to see him
three days dead. The river will have done
its work on him. And the fish. But drawn
by a soul-spun thread, compelled
to patch the jagged heart-hole, I drop
over the edge of the precipice, down
the shadowed canyon to its bouldered bed,
ear-stopping domain of torrent in flood.

His vessel, half-buried, a javelin
stuck against the flow, leads me
to him. But before the ropes can be applied
he washes free, slips between boulders, churns
through the drops and floats across
into the eddy next to me.

Cradled in my arms, how does he look?
I do not care. I stroke
his hair, tenderly caress the forehead
with its tiny bruise. And cling
when they come to me to say
"Enough," to what I cannot bear to leave.

We struggle to line him up the last pitch
to where his mother waits.
I cannot speak. I feel
my forever-part arrested
in mid-leap, astonished to the core,
still roped to him. My heart embroidered
with finely wrought stitches. Each one
sweats a tiny crimson drop.

■ 9-11

Just today, four days
after the attack, my eyes
tear up when Ray Charles sings
"America the Beautiful"
on oldies radio. I have to stop
the car. From sea to shining sea
we try to comprehend the world
has changed. Perhaps it takes
a jet-fuel inferno, 1600 degrees
to purge our petty hates, our
puerile road-rage. Soon
we'll have burned clean, bright
with resolve to change
the old world order. Pray
it is done with mercy
for the wide-eyed children.
Pray it is done with mercy.

LAST TO GO

Maybe I can live till one hundred and eight,
or forty-eight, or nine, by transplantation,
of, first up, my lungs, cloned from sputum wisely
stockpiled. Next I'll pay to replace the parts
that clog and fail, all but for this brain
I can ill afford to crack, for whom I
shall have to borrow from others money they
will be saving for themselves, I know it.
Their need I will allow as great: to find
someone to lose his mind, and then to die:
to keep alive the romance of the poet.

◼ MORNING IN THE BUSH

The currawongs advance
branch by branch.
Black wings slit the canopy
(sky blue, leaf green).
Glinting eyes try
to outstare the man
walking amongst their trees.

Black scythes slash the day.
Down pours that night:
wind-lashed trees drop flowers
like sobs for the life
you snatched away.

Koori woman,
stolen child,
where is my innocence?
Did you know I couldn't see
the suicide in your smile?

I hated death
as the young doctor should.
I thought I held you up.
I fell so hard.
Where were the tablets I gave you?
The books I read?

You cut me with your truth.
My grief was not for you.
Now the wind
is only cold, and I know
I don't belong, here,
amongst the trees
or the birds
that keep their careful distance.

▓ THE MUSE COLLAPSES

Lifting my lady's delicate hand
gazing into her bewildered eyes
I murmur "I'm sorry.
I know this will hurt"
then slap her veins hard at the wrist.
I watch her wincing,
weakening.

Her pulse is difficult to find.
Her heart's
alive
its rhythm
erratic.
Lying in a pool of blood
she needs some fluid yesterday.
I rip packets open,
ready an intravenous drip
but there's no one about to help.
"Damn and curses,
where are the nurses?"
I expostulate, to make conversation.
She looks at me blankly.

The woman has no poetry
in her blood.
I slap her again,
slip in a line,
squeeze the bag hard.

IDIOM

When her mind left her so did the world,
Having furnished a shrine
With long halls of mopped tiles
And pink rose wallpaper, the perfunctory
Young caretakers of an age.
                                        But now
And then while they clattered a spoon
Of gruel between her teeth or hoisted
Her naked on the shower chair, she'd blurt out
A tiny fragment of her life,
Saying *Henry, Henry, I see the lake*
Or *This is the music I love.*

She'd emerge from mist and stone silence
Like a Delphic priestess, her voice
Sudden and foreign to them
In the day room, miraculous
For its unknowable context, the gist
Of ninety years; and they'd ignore
How real she'd become.

She had no past to speak of
Except when she spoke. Her days
Droned on and on. They could listen
To themselves hum as she talked,
Refusing to imagine her
Hair light brown as in the photograph
Her infrequent daughter brought
Like a chrysanthemum saved
From October frost.
                                Yet they felt
What they heard. Her comments had flesh,
A thin veil easily bruised. And even

When she stopped, her body continued
To whisper, its breathing

A common expression, its heartbeat
A proverb, but in a dead language, cryptic
As an oracle, wise beyond words.

■ THE MILES

A man cuts down his wife with the back
Of one hand and then the other
Like a combine blade through soft winter wheat
Building the lovely sheaves that save Grangeville, Idaho,
Each year. He does it for her, for the cigarette
With which he catches her out among the cottonwoods
And breaks in half, thin as the trembling fingers
He leaves alone, and then draws her close and loves her
With the same earthy hands. He leads her inside
And talks to her like someone who feeds a jittery bird
Out of his palm and coos in the way he imagines
A bird might, telling her again
How his mother died of two gutted lungs, while he thinks
Of how his strong arms couldn't save her, holding her
So far above him in the little room upstairs,
Holding her back even as she cried out, even as her eyes
Fluttered so hard to rise into their own steady stare.
Sometimes closeness is wrong
Because it hides a thing's true distance
Like his voice from which she leans away
After they sprawl on the bed for a while,
Straightening her dress to spill smoothly
Over her marked body like a white muslin waterfall,
Or the Clearwater mountain range that looks so easy
From their back porch. Much closer, a few wild lilies
Confused and ravaged by heat, bow in a field of dust
Like someone who can hardly move bent in half
To corner sheets. After his truck rattles off
She walks out as she has many times
As far as that tattered screen door
Where she fills her eyes with the same peaks
And lights up, waiting for the sweet backfire

Of a cough. When she puckers to exhale, one long puff
Holds together in the still air like a gray wren
Who briefly flits among the parched lilies
Before vanishing to its full height
And using all the miles that it can.

Before the cigar, the green fatigues, he guns
A motorcycle through the jungles and mountains
He inherits, just a middle class kid
Easy riding South America for kicks,
Chrome spokes in revolution, biblical rain
And villages decrepit as the bodies
Of lepers, the snake oil economies
Of countries prescribed by banks, and then
The motorcycle breaks. But begging
Lifts, lying exposed in the backs of trucks,
Even on foot, even rafting the Amazon,
In places the only road, he keeps rambling
Pell-mell as an amnesiac out to discover
Himself, past and future intertwined
Like serpents on a caduceus. Just a doctor,
Or not quite, halfway through training,
Not yet having to choose between a first aid kit
And a crate of bullets, he tours the camp, greets
The untouchable peasants with his bare hands,
Nothing but bravado to heal them with,
The cheapest kind of faith. Lost in his twenties,
He'd rather lie around a tent shirtless
And suck the milk from coconuts, flirt
With nuns. But here the patients usurp his role
As prophet, their deformities bizarre
Though undeniable as Elisha's revelation
To the Syrian king that he must walk
Disrobed into water, bathe in the Jordan
Seven times, a path clear of privilege,
And the physician who rode shotgun with Fidel
Right into the UN continues his education.
In the way the nerve goes and leaves no pain
When the maiming begins, toes and fingers

Falling off, the poor live as they live
And don't know. The river simmers with lanterns
His last night. Everyone waves a numb farewell.
But cleansed with their squalor he feels
A little fire beneath his skin, drifts on.

THE BIRTH OF FLOWERS

Imagine the shock—
amid a vast expanse of conifer
and moss, homely liverwort and ginkgo—
when the first petals appear

supple and pink as unknown human flesh,
pushing aside ancient horsetail and fern,
hue almost electric against
the unending green and brown.

Imagine the first sepals parting
to reveal stamen, pollen-dusted pistil,
the fragrance and honey of sex
both lurid and intoxicating—
the dizzying perfume
of earth become a boudoir.

And then the rapid proliferation
of forms and varieties, teeming meadows
orange and red and purple-throated.
The coming of tubers and bulbs,
seeded and pitted fruits,
hermaphroditic orchids.

Scientists would have us believe
it's all genetics, natural selection, survival
of the fittest: but can't explain
the sudden appearance of flowers.
So fragile and so useless,
of no great purpose, no obvious advantage.

Yet somewhere in the mid-Mesozoic,
post-Jurassic era, as if from the dark
emptiness of a long winter, the first spring
came to the planet, eggshell white
tinged with purple streaks—
and a new world bloomed.

■ LABYRINTHITIS

Five months ago, the telephone
rang: a voice saying his father
was dead—a ruptured aneurysm
early Sunday morning
while he was in the garden
clipping roses.

Now there's a ringing
in his ears, the room spinning
when he turns, and he's beginning
to wonder if he's not becoming
his old man.

He fidgets on the exam table,
kneading palms, as I narrate
the inner ear's anatomy, how rhinovirus
upsets our bearings.

We went boating the week before,
the man says, *and he was fine.*

I silence myself to listen
to whatever he has to say, and imagine
how for five months the words   father   dead
must have looped inside him.

How they entered his ears like a pair of ravens
and flapped against his tympanums, began
a rippling inside each fluid spiral
and funneled deeper, deeper. No longer as words,
but as shadows of words, a hush
left for him to unravel.

▪ FETUS PAPYRACEOUS

Sometimes one of the twins dies
in utero, without his mother
ever knowing she'd been twice blessed.
Hungry for life, the living twin
will absorb his double and growing
compress him until all that's left
is a tiny shape made flat, a silhouette
of the life it once contained.
While the one child is born pink
and howling into his parents' arms,
the other remains a faint imprint
barely visible in the translucent web
of amniotic membranes—a fetal hieroglyph.
Some people believe twins have
only one soul between them.
If that's true, how many
of us are born half—
ignorant of our paper twin, the ghostly
shroud of an other self,
the blank page into which all
our imagined lives are written.

RONALD PIES

THE ALZHEIMER SONNETS

Apple blossoms and a robin's egg sky
as I climbed higher, dizzying me,
until a fleck of bark fell in my eye.
I remember clear and sharp how that tree
shook my arms off its bearish trunk,
and sent me spinning in free fall,
clawing the air before the final clump
my leaden body made. I crawled
across the yard in league with death,
though my child's mind didn't know it.
I choked back tears and caught my breath,
biting down the pain. I wouldn't show it
then, or now, as the words spin
out from my tangled brain—if ever they were in.

The barn swallows swooped low
as we made a sweaty clamor in the hay.
Our first lusting tumbled slow
and musky, morning to noon that day.
That was just before our wedding vows
and that first, unbidden birth.
If I could harvest consonants and vowels
the way I ploughed your riven earth
our first nude morning, I'd be pleased.
The doctors say I'm losing parts of me
with each plaque and tangle of disease,
but I won't feel it. I stay lanky and free
in your hay-kissed arms, where fifty years
pass in an eye-blink that knows no tears.

Some nights still, I hear the horses cry
and smell the fire scorch their manes.
Death leapt up in our stallion's eye
as I tugged and wrangled with his reins.
You did your best to keep the water
coming, hose down the house,

and get our son and daughter
safe away. I ran to douse
the sparks that harried our lawn,
until, at last, the wailing engines came.
These days, my smell is nearly gone
for fruits and flowers—but old flames
still come back. With luck, I'll catch the scent
that love's blaze makes permanent.

The doctors say some pinkish sludge
is what does you in. Gobs of amyloid
and twisted strands that just won't budge
from the brain. Pretty soon, a void
of neurons hangs like some old
moth-eaten sweater, where once
a solid weave of bold
thought reigned. Yet the soul hunts
for clues among the mind's gray runes,
and now and then finds some Rosetta
Stone of memory—an old Sinatra tune
that brings back spirit, if not the letter.
Love, these cells that wink out one by one
are not the song of all that we've become.

■ CRISIS

I've set aside
   my prescription pad
and analytic calm—
   dropped all pretense
of science:
   it's you and me now,
pressed cold
   against death's ribs.
I use
   what tricks I know
to keep you living
   through another bony night,
another flurry
   of final phone calls.
And you, as always, refuting life:
   denaturing love, companions, sex.
Well, you leave my office alive.
   That's as close
to certainty
   as our work gets.

■ WAITING

Now she's gone to other hands
Whom carefully, I hope,
Wisely, I pray,
Will tease her tissues,
Separating what must stay from what
Can go; we both, together, having
Said good-bye to organs and to cyst,
Said good-bye as well to each other,
Just in case, only never thinking,
Never facing,
Not going on together.

My hospital has tried to bend her intractable spirit, I note,
With instructions about coughs and bandages
And where she will go while I wait somewhere else.
They showed her movies and gave her articles to read.
I think I hear her telling them to wait,
She has another page to finish.

I wait for her return,
Weakened by this unreasonable attack.
Both of us, diminished.
I wait in the hospital waiting room
with other waiting families and
watch waiters watching me.
This hospital has changed,
no longer friend to me, it is foreign.
I am stranger here like all these others,
waiting, fearing, not at home.
Time goes slowly here.
Each minute has all its seconds.
And I think, hopefully, of things we'll do
and where we'll go and
how we met and what a
Dear person she is when she isn't
being mulish.

■ MOTHER TERESA, THE CARDIOLOGIST

Mother Teresa,
known for her great heart,
has been reincarnated.
Now she is a cardiologist,
a proud man
who knows that he
is God's gift
to humanity,
and has no compassion,
no empathy,
not even kindness.

He knows about BNP and Echos
and rushes in to stent anyone
whose insurance might pay
then golfs three times a week.

Mother Teresa seldom asks
why or what she is or what
it is all about.
And once so humble
she now scoffs at all those
who didn't choose
a lucrative specialty.

She is much more content
and no longer asks God
to help the poor,
but some days
she would like a little
assistance
in reaching par.

POEM (LONG OVERDUE) FOR MR. MEEK

Frederick Meek, as mild as the very name,
speaks to me with wheezed and rasping care.
Icy linoleum snickers on the floor;
there's always a tang of urine in the room.

His lungs are a monument to cigarettes.
Yet he will talk by the hour, as he did one day
of his wife who died of cancer years ago.
And showed me her photo, nibbled by the rats.

I don't believe he suffers much—no wild
and adolescent anguish. No, for his part
he'd choose this clenched and shuttered room, no hurt

except the quiet agony of small things:
the toe that hurts him when it rains, the chilled
and useless testicles and the botched lungs.

NEW SECURE PSYCHIATRIC UNIT

It's really very nice
they've done a lovely job
in the space available.

Clean as a new pin
in speckled gray and green
the plaster dust and red flex swept

as far as the door
on the last day by leg-pulling
men with echoing radios.

Ten secure rooms
with no hanging points
as far as we can tell.

Ready for the voices
the conviction of delusion
the striking out in fear

the new futures
angry spouses
and the weeping parents.

The complaints of the advocates and
the watching waiting Boards
the Opposition, Ombudsman and Coroner

about the position of the taps
and the standard of our care. Today
we are thinking only, they've done a lovely job.

■ THE FACE

Superficial muscles as orbicularis oculi and oris
procerus, zygomaticus major, zygomaticus minor
buccinator, corrugator supercilii, going down
to the muscles of mastication, the masseter
temporalis and the medial and lateral pterygoids.

The ophthalmic artery wriggles into infra- and
supra-orbital branches as the facial nerve splits
into zygomatic, mandibular and buccal branches
and the temporomandibular joint waits
beneath parotid gland, just before the ears.

Vena vorticosa, vitreous body and optic foramen
of the eye, and the stylohyoid and styloglossus
suspend the tongue from styloid processes
of the skull, the frontal, maxilla, sphenoid and
zygomatic bones. Beauty lies beneath the skin.

WORDS

At night, in my bed, a rip-shirted
world still breathes, its muscle
    matched to mine, its rhythm

in my back, one slow heart
unschooled and warm. Come
    inside, check your coat,

remove your shoes—or keep them,
it is so risky, the intonations, the accents,
    the manipulations of day, its

science and short sun, its voluptuous,
sudden moon. A moon so focused
    I recorded its holes, the few

mumblings it could give. I saw these
things and kept their answers.
    Study the scenes—

on-call, a night's receiving room,
the dead woman, her chest open,
    my hand inside. That was

the night I took back those
early sayings, their recommended lists
    and ready places.

That night I crawled down
from the stacks. I kicked Dr. Osler
    and opened his tie, finding

old Halsted, scalpel raised and in
my face. And later, with Blalock—
    we chewed opium and talked

about pain. Remember
these nights, the short tempered
    streets. I sleep with this

world and speak its words,
the unstuck, the found, sentences
　　pale and sweating, that

whole language of make-do
words, every syllable bare-chested,
　　beside me still and breathing.

■ GAY MEN'S VD CLINIC

And when he dropped his pants
I found there was no bedroom
        or even a bed.
Maybe this is why some of the nits,
      the worried ones, have gone mad,
           aghast at this nature—
a love of mobile homes,
      tiny trailers that weave and mat
           as earth moves,
canyons rip
      and plains form.

Tentacles of pubic hair
spring and weave in a heaven raining dry
      pinpoint piles of mother blood,
      tumbled dust and ivory ribbed cocoons.
Shells and dander fall,
         cobbling his underwear with rusty tiles,
      rolling with precision into cracks,
           along the seams.

All this, as if the social order in a henhouse,
      the gentility in the community urinal
and the decorum of a shower stall
      fuel gossip among a cult of tiny crabs,
      those sleepless members who must somersault
         at the thought of moving on,
must spit their eggs
      among the high wires, frantically
         crusting the sky
with brittle satellites.

In his sagging shorts, flaked
      scabs line the wrinkles
         as an anxious galaxy swarms
above, its pace so frantic
        each louse must
        know the slight space
        as home, the duration as joy.

■ SHIFTS

By 3 AM our unit's beyond coming or going, no
fluorescence, only bedside lamps and a voiceless
blue. It's an ICU sky, techs returning like comets,
you with your pressure falling into a range where
stars form so quickly we can't keep up with
the numbers.

Your nurse bandaged wet spots where skin
wouldn't hold. Your planets wept like blisters,
your heaven so swollen it had to give.
And as we sopped, you soaked through the world
we'd known, no family holding you down,
no orbiting lover.

     We knew someone was talking
below, of what a body shouldn't endure, how it might
linger in what has to be pain, that system.
     But you couldn't hear them, could you?
Not as your ankles turned to air, not as we dialed
the only number you left us, your voice answering
like so many dead keep doing these nights, your machine
implying you'd heard us all along.
        Or so we took it

when you said who you were, your name and not
your number. You simply thanked us for the call.
Nothing, no requests, just that empty heaven
we refused to fill, your machine running
as the sky rose, your bandages pulled, the heavens
quiet as our hands passed over.

ELSPETH CAMERON RITCHIE

GUN IN THE CLOSET

Mom hates it when Dad
cleans the barrel,
then aims his sights at
Aunt Jenn on the wall.

Can't study any more. Instead
I play Guns and Roses.
Dad's gone to Saudi.

Mom's at the bar with that man.
I wait at home alone.

The liquor cabinet
only holds Dubonnet now.
I drank the sherry.

The red paint in my bedroom
blisters lonely walls.
No one noticed that knife.

My dog was run over last week.
Mom said, "Anyway, he drooled."

I tried aspirin last week
after Tom laughed "No" to the dance.
It only made me vomit.

The house is silent.
Dad taught me how to shoot.

Mom's still not home.

■ CALL IT

Call it when it's over.
Call it when you're through.
Call it when the body lies
   Still as stone, heavily supine.
Call it the coda of the code.
Call it flat line, end of the line
   Straight on through.
Call it a life, call it a day.
Call it the period
   Ending life's sentence.
Call it what you will.
Just be prepared—nothing undone
   From the first cry to long silence—
To call it. The code ends,
   Not in defeat, but acknowledgment.
Call it like an umpire: make the right call.
Runner out, but safe at home.
Make sure it's called for:
   Appropriate, correct, solemn.
The calling to heal pulls you.
When the beats are gone, nothing left to do
But call it.

INCOMPATIBILITY

Doctor—blood for your patient was just returned from another operating room

I am stunned
the words mean this:
my patient received blood incompatible with his own

time expands, as before a storm
          leaves flutter helplessly
exposing veined undersides

I see the bag still attached to the blood set
drained of color

sinewaves saw their way across the screen

my god, it can't be

surgeons bend to the dissection

and time contracts, jagged, explosive, heraldic lightning
pressure-urine-name-on-bag-urine-wound-pressure
the pulse oximeter beats steadily, like freight cars passing
now, now, now, now

I feel he is under a death sentence
with timed poison
I think any moment now
the end of the train will appear around the bend

I tell surgeons, nurses
bend to the task
          fluids-mannitol-gases-pressure
          empty the urine tube, again

the winds begin to gather
trees start to talk their whipping language
any moment now blood cells will lyse
I steady myself before the storm
          feel brushstrokes of air from the passing train
and wait for the moment
          he begins to die.

▪ LOSS

Half a life ago
I knew so many, many
ways to remember.
No more.
No longer does a gauze-choked winter sun
or a round moon balancing on a rooftop
force me to inhale sharply
turn my head
close my eyes and
Halt—steeped in remembrances.
Now, perhaps a sigh echoes briefly.
You, my father, are so very far away.

And now, my husband—
I live in fear of a shattering
of a chasm opening and
our fingers
grasping
reaching to hold
slipping—

our union no match
for the swiftness of the parting.
I feel the tingling
before numbness
before paralysis.

Sunlight sifts through dappled trees.
You kiss our clasped hands.
The day is like any other.

ONE MORNING

a word mocked her
innocently Seussed her
bumpity bumped her
dim light ghostie

the word seemed so plain jane
too slumpy grumpy
for a sloe-eyed morning

how ridiculous—it couldn't be
rumpin' 'n jumpin'
glee of unleashed dogs

but no—there it was
stump clump
pirates on deck
crimp crump
wrinkle-mouth spinster

sump pump
sewer dump

the river before
the dry creekbed after

one morning
in the shower
fingers stumble

a word forms
its small weight

her tongue whispers

lump

▓ TWO MEN

Two men sit quietly in a room
between a dying woman.
Both men know that she's dying
because one has slept by her side
for twenty-seven years and he's never
seen her sleep so soundly. The other
man has turned her file to the page where
her usual doctor has written
FOR PALLIATION ONLY, and doesn't feel
he needs to read much more. Two men
sit on either side of a bed in which one person
is dying, and one of them asks if the other
needs anything. "I'm OK," is the only reply
that's given. But as if shaken out of a stupor,
the object of this concern asks
the other if the cancer that's killing his wife is
"one of those silent ones." The correct answer
to his question is "Yes," but saying this
won't make this pain bearable
and won't make more space in a bed already
crowded by a frail woman sleeping beside
the life that's gone before her.
So before a reply is offered
the morphine pump buzzes mechanically
in the artificial space between
this conversation and empties the only
easy answer into an unseen vein.

TRANSPLANT

The heart was harvested in Wisconsin and flown in by helicopter.
—Atlanta radio news

Within the green purpose of the room
there were ten beating hearts, but now are nine
who help the otherworldly pump assume
the flow of blood along the plastic line

by which the tenth now lives and has his being—
which is slow asleep, but dreams of moving,
of breathing on its own, of dimly seeing
its alien toes awake, all ten approving

the knitting of this widely opened chest—
where now there is no heart, but only pocket
until the circling mercy comes to rest
as neatly as an eye within its socket

and then the shock, the charmed expectant start,
the last astonished harvest of the heart.

◾ VISITATION

December 2001

At Serenity Gardens, winter
has surrounded us. My mother's room
is way too warm for me,

just right for her—with an extra sweater.
Outside, this uneasy year, her 93rd,
lurches through December.

She is surely serene in this place,
thanks to whatever goodness;
queen of the electronic piano.

Among my chief duties now
I have become her human calendar,
a stay against time, her reach for the past.

Each visit, we review the years.
We sit and we talk, fragile mother,
absent-minded son.

This afternoon, I assemble for her
some semblance of my long-dead
father, the only husband she had.

I tell her his story.
We study his photograph.
Do you remember him, I ask?

She looks again.
No, she answers, softly. No.
But isn't he good looking!

She smiles. I chuckle.
In the gathering dark,
we cry a bit together:

I for what she has forgotten,
she for what I remember.

AFTER THE CONCERT: A CONFESSION

It was that string quintet by Brahms:
in F—the one that starts *allegro*
then in the second movement suddenly

turns *grave ed appassionato*: Remember?
That second movement was so full
of grace, viola singing so, the cello

grave and joyful both at once.
And there we were, you and I,
side by side by thigh breathing together.

So in the finale, in the glory
of that last fugue, *allegro energico*, it was,
when all heaven was breaking loose

I want you to know

now that the concert is over
and you have gone back
to your love and I to mine

I want you to know

how much, there in the middle of it all,
right there in front of God and everybody
how much I wanted to

ask you to dance.

SAND CRAB

I recently walked along the bay
with my five-year-old nephew.
What are those little holes
with bubbles coming out?
he asked. Sand crabs, I said.
They hide under a thin layer
of sand to protect themselves.

Have you ever seen one?
he wanted to know. Yes,
I said, thinking of my first day
at the Washington V.A. Hospital.
A young man, age twenty-two
was hidden under a white sheet.
He was pale as a moonbeam,

and his mouth puckered
in and out with each breath.
He returned from Vietnam
with acute leukemia. His name
was Howard, I said
out loud. You're making
it up, my nephew laughed.

■ NOT GOD

I thought to delay the answer, camouflage
it, by waiting until he asked another
question. But he prefaced the question with

I know you're not God. This is commonly said
to me, second in frequency only to What
would you do if it was your father, or wife,

etc. I accept this statement of my undeity
to be rhetorical, a mechanism to permit me
to be imprecise, to use phrases like "it depends

upon many factors" and "a range of." But lately
I'm increasingly tempted to say, How do you know
I'm not God? What gives you such certainty?

Do you say this to your lawyer, accountant,
or mother-in-law? And, if I'm not God then why
ask me a question that only God can answer?

■ WHAT I AM

You ask me how I know.
    It's hard to say. It's not
something I could easily
    teach, like palpation
of an enlarged liver.

I couldn't describe it
    with precision, i.e.,
sixth nerve palsy, the sound
    of mitral stenosis. Still,
after fifteen years

it's unmistakable. A fine tremor
    of his eyebrow,
the skin below his chin
    like papier-mâché,
the way his shoulder

tilts back to the right.
    He has less than
a few months to live. I can't say
    it's vascular,
or neurologic, or even

cancer, which I see
    every day. I only know
it's progressive
    and irreversible. It's
what I am proficient at.

DAVID WATTS

THE DAY I SHOWED MY PENIS TO THE LADY DOCTOR

Do you want to take a look at it? I asked.
This was after we'd talked
about the other lesions
scattered over my body like paint-ball hits
in a lost cause.
She said she thought she'd better.

A spider bit it, I joked.
She looked skeptical so I whizzed it out,
but not before thinking this is part
of what it is to see a doctor
and realizing I had, after all,
no hesitations.

She was ready
in her rubber gloves and scientific eyes.
It was moist and tumid
from all the itching
and I bent it side to side
to show
the splotches all over.
I turned it,
twisting down to the red spot,
the place in the night
I couldn't resist.

She kept her gloves
in the ready position, quivering
in the air around it. She said
I should rub this salve all over it.
I said I was grateful
and put my little tubes of medicine
in my pocket.

Then we both left the room real fast.

▪ PHYSICAL EXAM

I have told her I will not
do a pelvic, so already
we are on better terms.

I have learned when best
to say this,
so as to ease her fears.

But she worries that I
will examine her breasts, perhaps
take too much pleasure
with beauty,
with softness . . . it's possible.

The truth is
unlike those I have loved
I do not remember the breasts
I examine. I didn't think
it would be this way,
but it is.

And I feel the opening
of possibility, it's just that
it goes unrecorded,
as if to honor
the unspoken agreement. Afterwards,

a transformation,
as if through this intimacy
we have become part
of each other,
protective of each other—Don't
misunderstand,
it's just that now
she stands close to me
and is not afraid.

■ APNEA

They said it was normal
for premature infants to stop breathing
sometimes.
And though I'm sure they meant to reassure
it didn't feel like comfort, exactly.
If I thought about it from a place
outside the moment
I might believe
he would be all right.
But to see this small baby
not breathing . . .

I said I was afraid
we hadn't done enough
to make him want
to live
in this place of raw light,
plastic isolettes,
oxygen streaming
through the silicon tubing.

So I sit beside him
and make small human noises
against the whir and whine
of intensive care:
I clear my throat,
clack my tongue,
I make those "Oh my soul" sounds
you understand in conversation
without making out the words.
I wrap my palm
around his rump
so he can feel
the warmth of my hand
claiming him,
rocking him slowly
into the family.

■ MY ID

April Wednesdays
my Id drives off for fishing.
His Chevy beater vetoes seat belts
unleaded gas, any tires but retreads.

All the way, a grin shimmies his lips.
He hums, Un-hunh un-hunh de duhnh de-dunh
halts his steed, disgorges from cavernous trunk guts
a rusty tackle box, three Budweisers
a folding K-Mart patio chair,

wipes mayo from his cheek,
trashes double-bacon-burger wrappers,
shovels pork rinds with a fist,
balances blood worms in Styrofoam cups
with plastic stick-on lids.

A fiberglass rod from childhood
snags blackberry bramble
by the mud-slicked bog near the lake.
He ignores a lawnmower's buzz, a
telephone's cry, an ambulance shriek.

Mute tree branches wave and wag in vain
to sign their message to a deaf universe.
Under skies like an overturned canyon,
that tease of a sudden drenching,
he fishes for just this moment.

As afternoon sun drains red to the lake
he reels in random red thoughts—
red dogs, red flannel hash browns
red wrappers from Tampa cigars.

He pictures his redheaded woman
as raspberry creamsicle
meltingly soft on a jade green plate,
guns the motor,
sprints his Impala home for dessert.

◼ MY SPEEDOMETER

Like a heart in fibrillation
the needle bounced with each bump—
shimmy wobble jolt bounce crump.
At 45th Street it struck zero, fell limp
as Old Bessie hummed around the bend.

I think it was broken long ago.
Never could cope with high speeds
always zooming too fast,
overexcited, nervous junior leaguer
shot air balls and bricks,
foul shots like chunks of dead wood
that thunked off the backboard.

Maybe that's why I'm suddenly happy
this morning at the keyboard,
since my speedometer has finally quit
from forever giving me
that pokey orange finger. After all,

there are places to go where speed
is not measured in miles per hour
and at some point I finally do need
to discover the pace
that will carry me swiftly
but not crazily
into the shrink-wrapped future.

■ BLEED

I had just come to the chapter
about your disease.
I was reading about it.
I had learned some things
staying up all night while
a young mother vomited blood.
I looked things up later,
after the priest refused to come
to a Jewish hospital.
Her sisters and I
invented our own last rites.
No one had known she drank.
I lay on the top bunk
in the call room at 3 A.M.
reading the list of symptoms.
I understood. I thought of you.

KINDERGARTEN PHYSICAL

6th of 8 children
he stands,
stripped to his superman
underwear,
round scars on chest
and back,
one thick straight scar
(razor cut)
down the trunk,
and, removing his sock
the ring:
"Mama use to chain me
down the basement."

■ HEART SOUNDS

The doctor moved his stethoscope
along the rib cage
to the outermost edge of her breast

where he could hear the extra sounds
above and beyond
simple valve openings and closures
the asymmetric chorus
the ragged ejection
     of clicks rubs claps
     leaks and murmurs
the vortex as the ventricle
     filled and
     squeezed
     and with a sudden thunderous expulsion
     collapsed the cavity
     to a serenade
of reverberations and echoes.

She remembered

     holding her breast
     slightly up
     like this,

     to reach another's lips

then felt the paper sheet beneath her
let the breast sag to the side

let him do to her as he would
let him hear whatever he wished.

▪ MY TOMOGRAPHY REPORT

It's not like I need,
at seventy-two,
continuous denial of death.

Actually, knowing it will be my heart,
that most common of doors,
comes with relief.

Still, I did expect when the news came
clarification would begin:
contrast between greens sharper,
yellows turn golden, white
suddenly transparent.

But no:

Edges of tree shadows
moving across my spring lawn remain silent;
horns in the andante of Mahler's *Ninth*
still only distant calling;
those I hold close, no closer.

The only differences:
three pill bottles lined up
behind my Listerine toothpaste,
a spray vial of nitroglycerine (just in case)
in my keys-pocket,

and these annoying rumors
whispering along the dark alleys
of my chest.

■ THE OTHER MAN *IS* ME

for Benny Williams

> . . . *the word was made flesh*
> *and dwelt among us . . .*

It happens, rarely
—like an epiphany:
a word dances off the page
clothed in its finest attire
lifting your eyes,
or it shouts within an utterance
turning your head.

But, mostly, words in dictionaries
line up, dry bones in a box.
Take the word *grace*:
dictionaries don't show grace
leading a stubborn man to goodness;
or *humane*:
the dictionary ordains it
benevolent, merciful, kind.
For murder, cruelty, rape,
as if naming a separate species, *in*
is prefixed to the word.

But bless you Benny
when you say about a friend,
concerning her cruel husband,
She's accepted his humanity,
instantly,
grace and humanity dance together,
watering my bones.

Even today, nine days later,
when Timothy McVeigh is executed
for bombing the Federal building
in Oklahoma City, killing 168
men, women and children,

the way you uttered his humanity
—from the darkened back seat
as we drove home from Pork Pie:
A Jazz Legend—so matter-a-fact-ly,
the reach of it still, strangely,
comforts me.

■ WHITE ROSE

White rose, white rose,
three summers I've watched you eke
existence on a strip of hardpan
pinched on one edge by basalt,
on the other, by a concrete alley.

How did you get here,
crowded by curb-to-curb parking?
Daytime shoppers on their way to bookstores
and boutiques in Pioneer Square
don't loll to praise. Nighttime visitors like me
hurry downhill to ball games, home shows,
boat shows, dirt bike races, monster truck drags,
a rose the last thing on our minds.

If planted to soften ugliness or salve
the conscience of an absentee-owner
it was a mistake: you are not lovely,
you smell of exhaust.
Your irrigation system: run-off
through oil seep.
Food? Mulching? I have no idea.
To add insult: beer and wine bottles
strewn in your gangly brambles.

My guess is, you were abandoned.
Perhaps when an owner cleared out,
unable to make taxes on this prime
southwest-sloping property.
Then, surrounded by the fragrance,
the bright colors of related flowers,

you produced a profusion of blooms
double the size of the tattered skirt
you wear tonight as I walk by
on my way to the car,
past the Yesler Street viaduct,
beneath which the homeless
make their beds.

■ HUTALA, AFGHANISTAN

A child is not a lion, is not, is not a zero.
Collateral damage can never, never be
excused or written off as just an accident.
The tiny shoes, the braided caps displayed
on the dirt mounds. The grief like a nail
hammered into the skull and no way to pull
it out. Seven boys and two girls and one
young man, about to be married, gone,
gone forever. And the pilot whose rocket
exploded their lives, staring in the dark.
Don't blame God. It's not his fault. Blame
us all. We forgot, children are flowers.

Perhaps it was the howls
from the kennels, or the merciless insomnia
that grips men of thought, but that night Louis Pasteur had a frightful
dream that his little patient, Joseph Meister, was dying.

He knew the symptoms, having witnessed them himself as a boy in Arbois.

The snapping jaws, foam-flecked, the slobbering bite.
Then the clumsy attempt at treatment,
cauterization at the smithy with a red-hot iron, screams,
the smell of burning flesh.
And inevitably, later, the faint tingling in the cicatrix,
the suffocation at the very sight of water,
the paralysis, the coma and death, always the death.

He woke to the wind scratching at the window like a dog.

But had he not been careful? . . . Trephining the skulls
of dogs, inoculating infected tissue under their scarlet brain-caps;
the transfer to rabbits, their spinal cords
hanging in flasks, shriveling, like tiny criminals on the gallows;
then turning the evil
back on itself by injecting it into infected dogs . . . who lived!

Light came, the lion, to the grounds of Villeneuve l'Etang.

And that day, July 6, 1885, Joseph, age nine, hands, legs, thighs
purple with bites from a rabid dog,
would become the first to receive the injections
of the rabbit spinal cord into the skin of his abdomen,
crying at first, then
submitting quietly under the watchful eyes of "dear Monsieur Pasteur."

What do we do in the face of evil?
Consider the exact arc that curved from Arbois to Paris.

And consider this . . .
fifty-five years later, on June 14, 1940, a sad day for the "City of Light,"

the knock of a rifle-butt on a gate, and the gatekeeper
who would commit suicide to avoid opening Pasteur's burial crypt to the
  Nazis.
That gatekeeper's name was Joseph Meister.

■ EMERSON'S APHASIA

Nature . . . disdains words . . . yet solicits the pure in heart to draw on all its omnipotence.
—from his essay "Fate"

In the carriage down from Concord, 1879—

one wheel bounces over a pothole
and a skeletal hand reaches out to grip the open window.

Then a distant thunder-clap
as the gold flood of sunlight shuts off.

"The- the- the- How do you call what stores up water
till it suddenly- suddenly- what shall I say?
Not squeezed out."

"A sponge," the other passenger suggests.
"No, no," with the sweetest of smiles and a sweeping
motion of his other hand up to the sky.

"The clouds perhaps?" is the next suggestion.

"Yes, the clouds are rolling up."

The carriage lurches and it starts to rain, the drops like bites
of a tiny kitten on the back of his hand.

"Shall I close the window?" the passenger asks.

"No," comes the answer. "No, no, no!"

Dannie Abse was born in Wales in 1925. He spent many years as a chest specialist in a London teaching hospital. He has published some twenty books, including four novels and a memoir. *White Coat, Purple Coat: Collected Poems 1948–1988* was published in the United States in 1993. His two most recent books are *Be Seated, Thou* (2000) and *The Yellow Bird* (2004).

Sharon Balter is an internist and epidemiologist who currently works for the Bureau of Communicable Disease at the New York City Department of Health and Mental Hygiene.

Iain Bamforth completed his training as a general practitioner in rural Scotland, an experience that is reflected in both of the poems selected for this edition. His fourth collection of poetry, *A Place in the World*, appeared in 2005. His interest in cultural issues, including the history of medicine, and in Europe's communities and languages, are expressed in his *A Body in the Library* and in his collection of essays *The Good European*, to be published at the end of 2006.

Angela Belli is professor of English at St. John's University in New York. She is the author of *Ancient Greek Myths and Modern Drama: A Study in Continuity*, coeditor of *Blood and Bone: Poems by Physicians*, and editor of the forthcoming *Bodies and Barriers: Dramas of Dis-ease*. Her scholarly interests focus on modern drama and on literature and medicine. She has served as chair of the English Department at St. John's University and as president of the New York College English Association.

Richard Berlin received his undergraduate and medical education at Northwestern University. His first collection of poems, *How JFK Killed My Father*, won the Pearl Poetry Prize 2002. Berlin also writes poetry for a monthly column, "Poetry of the Times," in the *Psychiatric Times*. He is an associate professor of psychiatry at the University of Massachusetts Medical School where he has established a creative writing award for medical students. He practices psychiatry in a small town in the Berkshire hills of western Massachusetts.

Paul Boor lives on Galveston Island where he is a pathologist, scientist, and teacher at the University of Texas Medical Branch. His poetry has appeared since 1976 in such places as *Rhino, Sulphur River, Journal of Medical Humanities*, and *Exquisite Corpse*. His short stories have been published in *Puerto del Sol, Mediphors, New Mexico Humanities Review*, and *Hardboiled*.

A native of Brooklyn, **George Braman** is assistant professor in the Department of Preventive Medicine and Community Health at the State University of New York, Downstate Medical Center, and currently teaches in the department's Master of Public Health Program. His experience includes seven years as public health physician with the New York State Department of Health and clinical and teaching positions in geriatric medicine. His interests encompass medical ethics and poetry. Several of his poems have been published in the *Annals of Internal Medicine*.

Richard Bronson is professor of obstetrics and gynecology at the Health Sciences Center, SUNY Stony Brook. He is on the board of the Long Island Poetry Collective, an editor of their literary magazine, *Xanadu*, and has been a featured reader for the Performance Poets Association. He is the 2003 recipient of the poem of the year award of the American College of Physicians.

Daniel C. Bryant grew up in Cincinnati, graduated from Princeton and Columbia, and practiced general internal medicine in Portland, Maine, until his retirement in 1999. His poetry and stories have appeared in numerous medical and literary journals, including the *Bellevue Literary Review*. In 2005 he donated his large collection of books by physician-writers to the Ehrman Medical Library at New York University Medical Center.

Catherine V. Caldicott is a faculty member in the Center for Bioethics and Humanities, SUNY Upstate Medical University, Syracuse. In addition to teaching ethics, she conducts empirical research on moral decision-making among medical students and physicians.

Rafael Campo teaches and practices general internal medicine at Harvard Medical School and Beth Israel Deaconess Medical Center in Boston. He is the author of *The Other Man Was Me* (1994), which won the 1993 National Poetry Series award; *What the Body Told* (1996), which won a Lambda Literary Award for Poetry; *Diva* (1999); and *Landscape with Human Figure* (2002). A Guggenheim scholar, Campo has published collections of essays including *The Poetry of Healing* (1997) and *The Healer's Art* (2003).

Robert Carroll is a psychiatrist in private practice in Los Angeles and a poet. He is on the clinical faculty in the Department of Psychiatry at UCLA and teaches family psychiatry at Cedars-Sinai Medical Center. He has published articles, poems, stories, and chapters in the psychiatric, medical, and poetry literatures and is the author of many chapbooks of poetry. He was a member of the Los Angeles Performance Poetry Slam Team for three years. He currently serves as vice president for institutional outreach for the National Association for Poetry Therapy.

Ron Charach is a practicing psychiatrist and the author of seven poetry collections. His *Selected Poems: Life in the Late Hours* will be published in late 2007. Charach lives in Toronto with his wife, Alice, a psychiatric researcher, and their two grown children.

A graduate of Georgetown Medical School, **Patrick Clary** is medical director of the only freestanding nonprofit hospice in New Hampshire and is board certified in family practice and hospice and palliative medicine. His poems have appeared in the *New England Journal of Medicine*, *CoEvolution Quarterly*, *Patient Care*, *Journal of Palliative Medicine*, and *Journal of Medical Humanities* as well as in anthologies, literary magazines, and three collections, most recently *Catch & Release* (2006).

Jack Coulehan directs the Institute for Medicine in Contemporary Society at Stony Brook University. His *The Medical Interview: Mastering Skills for Clinical Practice* (fifth edition, 2006) is a best-selling text on the clinician-patient relationship. He edited *Chekhov's Doctors* (2003), a collection of Chekhov's medical tales, and coedited *Blood and Bone: Poems by Physicians* (1998). His poetry and stories have appeared in medical and literary magazines in the United States, Canada, Australia, and the United Kingdom. *Medicine Stone* (2002) is the most recent of his four collections of poetry.

Richard Donzé is a physician board certified in preventive medicine and a published poet, essayist, and author. His work appears regularly in *JAMA* and other medical and lay publications, and several pieces were included in two collections of physician poetry (*Blood and Bone* and *Uncharted Lines*). In addition to his primary responsibilities at the Chester Hospital in West Chester, Pennsylvania, Donzé is also a faculty member at the University of Phoenix Online.

Thomas Dorsett has been practicing pediatrics for over thirty years. He is the author of one poetry collection and two volumes of translated poetry. Over the past three decades, examples of his poetry have appeared in over four hundred journals. He has also published numerous essays and translations.

Kirsten Emmott was born in Edmonton, Alberta. She is the mother of two children and lives in Comox, British Columbia, where she practices as a family doctor. Her most recent book is *How Do You Feel?* (1992).

D. A. Feinfeld attended the University of Rochester and Columbia University College of Physicians and Surgeons. His poetry has appeared in *Ploughshares*, *Atlanta Review*, *The Hollins Critic*, *JAMA*, and *Annals of Internal Medicine*. He is the author of three collections of poems: *What Do Numbers Dream Of?* (1997), *Bestiary Of The Heart* (2000), and *Rodin's Eyes* (2004). Feinfeld practices and teaches nephrology at Beth Israel Medical Center in New York City.

Serena Fox is an internist and critical care specialist in Washington, D.C. She works with refugees seeking asylum in the United States as a member of the Asylum Network of Physicians for Human Rights. Her poems have appeared in leading medical and literary magazines including *Poetry*, *JAMA*, and *Paris Review*.

Jerome W. Freeman, a practicing physician and educator, is on the faculty of the University of South Dakota School of Medicine and Augustana College. He has a particular interest in biomedical ethics and the use of literature for teaching about illness, the patient, and the caregiver. He has published three volumes of poetry and a collection of essays.

Arthur Ginsberg is a neurologist and poet based in Seattle. He has published in many poetry and medical journals. His work appears in the anthology *Blood and Bone* and his book, *Walking the Panther*, was published in 1984. He was awarded the William Stafford prize in 2003 by the Washington Poets Association.

Peter Goldsworthy divides his time equally between writing and medicine. He has won major literary awards across many genres. His most recent bestselling novel, *Three Dog Night*, won the Fellowship of Australian Writers 2004 Christina Stead Award. His works have been translated into numerous Asian and European languages. He has been awarded the Commonwealth Poetry Prize and the Australian Bicentennial Poetry Award. Three of his novels are currently being adapted for the screen and three for the stage.

John Graham-Pole is professor of pediatrics, medical director of Shands Arts in Medicine, and medical director of Pediatric Hospice of North Central Florida. He has authored or edited five books and made a CD of original poetry and music. He is well known nationally and internationally for his presentations on holistic medicine, palliative care, humor, and the healing arts.

Jennifer Harrison is an Australian poet and child psychiatrist. She runs the Developmental Assessment Program at the Alfred Hospital in Melbourne, Victoria. Her three poetry collections include: *Michelangelo's Prisoners* (winner of the 1995 Anne Elder Award); *Cabramatta/Cudmirrah*; and *Dear B*. In 2003 she won the NSW Women Writers National Poetry Prize and in 2004 was awarded the Martha Richardson Poetry Medal. Her poetry has appeared in *The Best Australian Poetry 2003*, *The Best Australian Poems 2004*, and will feature in *The Best Australian Poetry 2005*.

Norbert Hirschhorn is a physician specializing in the public health of women, children, and communities in the United States and the Third World. In 1993 he was commended by President Bill Clinton as an "American Health Hero." In 1994 Hirschhorn received a master in fine arts degree from Vermont College. His poems have been published in over a dozen journals and three anthologies. A chapboook of poems, *Renewal Soup*, was published in 1996 and a full volume, *A Cracked River*, in 1999.

Alice Jones's books include *The Knot*, *Isthmus*, *Anatomy*, and *Gorgeous Mourning*. Her poems have appeared in *Ploughshares*, *Colorado Review*, *Poetry*, and *Harvard Review*. Her awards include the Robert H. Winner award from the Poetry Society of America and an NEA fellowship. After working in internal medicine, she now practices psychoanalysis and is a training and supervising analyst at the San Francisco Psychoanalytic Institute.

Chuck Joy completed medical school at the University of Pittsburgh in 1978. He practices community child and adolescent psychiatry. The author of *Where We Will Go* (1995) and *How to Feel* (2005), he addresses character, relationships, and meaning in his poems.

Herbert Krohn grew up in inner-city Newark, New Jersey, and has practiced emergency medicine at Bellevue and Harlem hospitals and presently at Massachusetts General Hospital in Boston. His poems based on his Vietnam War experiences received national attention in the 1970s. His jazz quartet, Blue Cabaret, plays in the Boston area. He lives with his wife, Harriet Rosenstein, in Brookline, Massachusetts.

Michael Lieberman is director of the Methodist Hospital Research Institute and chair of the Department of Pathology at the Methodist Hospital in Houston, Texas. He has published four volumes of poetry. A fifth collection, tentatively titled *Unholy Vessels*, is out for review. He and his wife live in Houston and have two grown children.

Wayne Liebman is a playwright and poet. Among his honors are first place in the Maxim Mazumdar Playwriting Competition, second place in the Sprenger Lang Foundation's U.S. History Play Competition, and a New Play Production Grant from the National Foundation for Jewish Culture. Liebman is the author of *Tending the Fire* and coedited *Raising the Roof*, an anthology of poems for Habitat for Humanity.

Beth Lown, a general internist based in Boston and Harvard Medical School, began to write poems about her patients as a medical intern and has continued to write about, with, and for her patients, students, residents, and fellow learners. Her areas of interest and responsibility include faculty development in medical education, teaching and research in communication skills, and the relational aspects of care.

Ted McMahon is a Seattle pediatrician and poet. He currently practices half-time in the Seattle neighborhood of Ballard and devotes the other half to writing and to leading river journeys. His poetry has appeared in journals including *Seattle Review, Convolvulus, Manzanita Quarterly, JAMA,* and others. In 1999 he received the Carlin Aden Award for formal verse from the Washington Poets Association. He is a coeditor of Floating Bridge Press, publishing the work of Washington State poets. McMahon published his full-length collection of poetry, *The Uses of Imperfection,* in 2003. In 2004 he was awarded a Washington State Artist Trust Grant.

Tim Metcalfe graduated in medicine in 1984 and literature in 1995, has worked as a flying doctor and a soapmaker, and currently works full-time on poetry. His third collection, *Into the No Zone*, was highly commended in the 2004 ACT Publisher's Awards. He brings poetry to medical students at Australian National

University and is poetry editor of *Australian Family Physician*. He has promoted poetry on community radio since 1991.

David Moolten was born in Boston in 1961. His poems have been widely published and anthologized and his first book, *Plums & Ashes*, won the Samuel French Morse Poetry Prize in 1994. His second book, *Especially Then*, was published in 2005. A practicing pathologist with special expertise in transfusion medicine, Moolten works for the American Red Cross in Philadelphia, where he also lives with his wife and two daughters.

Peter Pereira is a family physician at High Point Community Clinic in West Seattle, where he takes care of an urban underserved population. Many of his poems arise from his medical practice and have appeared in *Poetry*, *Prairie Schooner*, *Virginia Quarterly Review*, *JAMA*, and elsewhere. He presented from his work at the first-ever "Vital Lines, Vitals Signs" poetry and medicine conference at Duke University Medical School in 2004. His books include *The Lost Twin* (2000) and *Saying the World* (2003), which won the Hayden Carruth Award.

Ronald Pies is clinical professor of psychiatry at Tufts University School of Medicine in Boston. Pies has published poetry in *JAMA*, *Literary Review*, *Connecticut River Review*, and other journals. He is the author of a collection of poems, *Creeping Thyme* (2004), and a collection of short stories, *Zimmerman's Tefillin* (2004). He is also the author of *Ethics of the Sages*, a work on comparative religious ethics, and several psychiatric textbooks.

Frederic Platt is a general internist in practice in central Denver since 1970. He has written extensively, including *Case Studies in Emergency Medicine*, now in its third edition, and three books about medical communication, *Conversation Failure* (1991), *Conversation Repair* (1995), and *The Field Guide to the Difficult Patient Interview* (second edition, 2004). He is also a poet.

Craig Powell was born in Wollongong in 1940 and raised in Sydney. A practicing psychiatrist and psychoanalyst, he moved to Canada in the 1990s. He is the author of eight books of poetry, of which the latest is *Music and Women's Bodies* (2002).

Saxby Pridmore is a professor of psychiatry at the University of Tasmania, Australia. He also has specialist qualifications in public health, pain medicine, and addiction medicine. He has written medical textbooks and over two hundred published poems. He lives in Hobart, Tasmania, with his wife, Mary, and son, William.

Dwaine Rieves, an intensive care physician, works as a volunteer in the VD Clinic of Whitman-Walker Clinic in Washington, D.C. His poems have appeared in *Georgia Review*, *Virginia Quarterly Review*, and *River Styx*.

Elspeth Cameron Ritchie trained at Harvard, George Washington, Walter Reed, and the Uniformed Services University of the Health Sciences. Her assignments have taken her to Korea, Somalia, Israel, Iraq, and Vietnam. Currently she is the psychiatry consultant to the U.S. Army Surgeon General. She is an internationally recognized expert in the management of disaster and combat mental health issues. She also has published poetry in numerous journals, focusing on the military, medicine, and mental health.

Bonnie Salomon is an emergency physician in the Chicago area. Her poems and essays have appeared in *The Lancet, Annals of Internal Medicine, The Pharos,* the *Chicago Tribune,* as well as several anthologies. She also teaches medical ethics to undergraduates at Lake Forest College.

Audrey Shafer is an associate professor of anesthesia at Stanford University School of Medicine and the Veterans Affairs Palo Alto Health Care System. She directs the Arts, Humanities, and Medicine Program through the Stanford Center for Biomedical Ethics. She is the author of *Sleep Talker: Poems by a Doctor / Mother* (2001) and a children's novel, *The Mail Box,* forthcoming.

Shen is a general practitioner in Adelaide, South Australia. He has published and performed widely. His most recent book of poems is *City of My Skin* (2001).

John Stone, a cardiologist, is emeritus professor of medicine and former associate dean for admissions at Emory University School of Medicine. He has published five books of poetry, the most recent of which is *Music from Apartment 8: New and Selected Poems* (2004). He is also the author of *In the Country of Hearts* (1993), a book of essays and stories, and coeditor with Richard Reynolds of the anthology *On Doctoring* (third edition, 2001).

Marc J. Straus, formerly chief of oncology at New York Medical College, practices medical oncology in White Plains, New York. He is the author of *One Word* (1994), *Symmetry* (2000), and *Not God* (2006), a poem-play that has been produced off-Broadway. He has published widely in poetry journals including *Kenyon Review, Field, Ploughshares,* and *Triquarterly* and has authored nearly one hundred scientific publications.

David Watts's early training was as a musician, then as a doctor. He practices medicine and gastroenterology and teaches at the University of California at San Francisco. His books of poetry include *Taking the History, Making,* and *Slow Waking at Jenner-by-the-Sea.* He is a regular commentator on National Public Radio's *All Things Considered* and holds a number of national media awards. His *Bedside Manners,* a collection of medical stories, was published in 2005.

Karl Weyrauch, from Seattle, is a family physician on the staff of the Western Institutional Review Board. He edits *eZAAPP,* an international weekly poetry zine for medical providers. His poetry has been nominated for a Pushcart

Prize and has appeared in *JAMA, Rosebud, Texas Observer*, and many others. His latest projects include a poetry video, "Zapped," and a movie screenplay, "Dueling Dynamos."

A New Hampshire native, **Kelley Jean White** studied at Dartmouth College and Harvard Medical School and has been a pediatrician in inner-city Philadelphia for more than twenty years. Her poems have been widely published over the past five years, including several book collections and chapbooks, and have appeared in numerous journals including *Exquisite Corpse, Nimrod, Poet Lore, Rattle*, and *JAMA*.

Born in Nebraska, **Robert Harlan Wintroub** received his education in Michigan, Nebraska, Oxford, and in Los Angeles. Clinical professor of medicine at UCLA, he began writing poetry in 1990, publishing in *Onthebus*. In the last ten years, he has emerged as a sculptor and has exhibited work in New York, Brookgreen Sculpture Garden in South Carolina, and in California.

John Wright is clinical professor emeritus at the University of Washington. He practiced internal medicine and endocrinology in Seattle from 1964 to 1994, during which time he held the position of medical director at the Swedish Medical Center. His poems and short stories have appeared in *JAMA, Annals of Internal Medicine, Journal of Family Practice*, and *Bulletin of the King County Medical Society*.

George Young practiced internal medicine and rheumatology at the Boulder Medical Center in Boulder, Colorado, from 1970 to 2002. He has been widely published in medical journals and literary magazines. A full-length collection of his poems, *Spinoza's Mouse*, won the 1996 Washington Prize in Poetry.

PERMISSIONS

Abse, Dannie. "Among a Heap of Stones" from *The Yellow Bird*, Sheep Meadow Press, 2004, reprinted courtesy of the publisher. "A Doctor's Register" and "Refugee" from *Be Seated, Thou*, Sheep Meadow Press, 2000, reprinted courtesy of the publisher.

Balter, Sharon. "Advice to a First-Year Medical Student," used with permission of the poet.

Bamforth, Iain. "Scant Resources" and "A Shining" from the sequence "Doing Calls on the Old Portpatrick Road" in *Open Workings*, Carcanet Press, 1996, reprinted courtesy of the publisher.

Berlin, Richard. "How JFK Killed My Father," "Piano Music," and "Radium Girls" from *How JFK Killed My Father*, Pearl Editions, 2004, reprinted courtesy of the poet.

Boor, Paul. "Blood Song," *Journal of Medical Humanities* 22.4 (2001): 301–302, reprinted courtesy of the publisher.

Braman, George. "Entitlements," *Journal of Medical Humanities* 25.3 (2004): 232, reprinted courtesy of the publisher.

Bronson, Richard. "Plague Doctor," *Journal of Medical Humanities* 24.1/2 (2003): 162–163, reprinted courtesy of the publisher.

Bryant, Daniel C. "Nursing Home," *Journal of Medical Humanities* 22.3 (2001): 209, reprinted courtesy of the publisher.

Caldicott, Catherine V. "Radiology," *Journal of Medical Humanities* 25.2 (2004): 153, reprinted courtesy of the publisher.

Campo, Rafael. "What I Would Give" and "Questions for the Weather" from *Landscape with Human Figure*, Duke University Press, 2002, reprinted courtesy of the publisher; "The Cardiac Exam" from *Diva*, Duke University Press, 1999, reprinted courtesy of the publisher.

Carroll, Robert. "Show and Tell" from *What Waiting Is*, In Corpus Press, 1998, reprinted courtesy of the poet.

Charach, Ron. "The Old Cardiology Dream" and "'In Panic as Killers Close In'" from *Elephant Street*, Signature Editions, 2003; "Hal" from *Petrushkin*, Ekstasis Editions, 1999, reprinted courtesy of the poet.

Clary, Patrick. "Five Tasks," *Journal of Medical Humanities* 22.1 (2001): 87–89, reprinted courtesy of the publisher; "Acute Myocardial Infarction," *New England Journal of Medicine* (November 19, 1981), reprinted courtesy of the publisher.

Coulehan, Jack. "Do No Harm," *JAMA* 292.22 (2004): 2698, reprinted courtesy of the publisher; "Phrenology," *Rattle* 9.1 (2003): 34, reprinted courtesy of the poet; "That Intern Dream," *Annals of Internal Medicine* 144 (2006): 308, reprinted courtesy of the publisher.

Donzé, Richard. "Four Perfect Quarters," JAMA 289 (2003): 1476, reprinted courtesy of the publisher.

Dorsett, Thomas. "Trisomy 13," *Journal of Medical Humanities* 22.3 (2001): 209, reprinted courtesy of the publisher. "On a Wizardless Ward," used with permission of the poet.

Emmott, Kirsten. "Anatomy," used with permission of the poet.

Feinfeld, D. A. "Itch" from *Bestiary of the Heart*, Fithian Press, 2000. First published in *Annals of Internal Medicine* 128 (1998): 305, reprinted courtesy of the publisher.

Fox, Serena. "Another Drive-By," *Paris Review* 161 (2002), reprinted with permission of the poet.

Freeman, Jerome W. "Carrying On" from *Starting from Hear: Dakota, Poetry, Pottery, and Caring*, Ex Machina Press, 1996, reprinted courtesy of the poet. "The Trojans," used with permission of the poet.

Ginsberg, Arthur. "Benign Fasiculations," JAMA 291 (2004): 2918 and "Epithalamium," JAMA 289 (2003): 1214, reprinted courtesy of the publisher.

Goldsworthy, Peter. "Suicide on Christmas Eve" and "Ode to Alcohol" from *This Goes with That*, ABC Enterprises, 1988, reprinted courtesy of the poet.

Graham-Pole, John. "Health Care" and "Last Rites" from *Quick*, Writers Club Press, 2002. "Health Care" first appeared in *Journal of Emergency Medicine* 12 (1994): 407, reprinted courtesy of the publisher.

Harrison, Jennifer. "Aus-Lan" from *Michelangelo's Prisoners*, Black Pepper Press, 1994, reprinted courtesy of the publisher.

Hirschhorn, Norbert. "Cambodians Celebrate the Buddhist New Year Once Again" and "Tuscan Still Life, with Sheep" from *A Cracked River*, Slow Dancer Press, 1999, reprinted courtesy of the poet.

Jones, Alice. "Expunge" and "Elide" from *Gorgeous Mourning*, Apogee Press, 2004, reprinted courtesy of the poet.

Joy, Chuck. "What If Lashika?" *The Pharos* 62 (1999): 8, reprinted courtesy of the publisher; "Blues for Me," *Cotyledon* 29 (2003): 2, reprinted courtesy of the poet.

Krohn, Herbert. "Bellevue Hospital Blues" and "True History of Orpheus" from *To Master Plan at the Crossroads*, Heron Press, 2004, reprinted courtesy of the poet.

Lieberman, Michael. "Pledge" and "Time to Depart" from *Remnant*, Sheep Meadow Press, 2002, reprinted courtesy of the poet.

Liebman, Wayne. "Monopoly," *Spillway*, reprinted courtesy of the poet.

Lown, Beth. "Home Visit," *Journal of Medical Humanities* 23.3/4 (2002): 264–265, reprinted courtesy of the publisher.

McMahon, Ted. "Silver Fork, American River" and "9-11" from *The Uses of Imperfection*, Cat 'n Dog Productions, 2003, reprinted courtesy of the poet.

Metcalfe, Tim. "Morning in the Bush" and "The Muse Collapses" from *Cut to the Word*, Ginninderra Press, 2002; "Last to Go" from *Into the No Zone*, Ginninderra Press, 2003, reprinted courtesy of the poet.

Moolten, David. "Idiom," *Poetry Northwest*, and "The Miles," *New England Review*, reprinted courtesy of the poet; "Che Guevara at the San Pablo Leper Colony, 1952," *Journal of Medical Humanities* 25.1 (2004): 67–68, reprinted courtesy of the publisher.

Pereira, Peter. "Fetus Papyraceous," "Labyrinthitis," and "The Birth of Flowers" from *Saying The Word*, Copper Canyon Press, 2003, reprinted courtesy of the poet.

Pies, Ronald. "Crisis" and "The Alzheimer Sonnets" from *Creeping Thyme*, Brandylane Publishers, 2004. "The Alzheimer Sonnets" were first published in *JAMA* 286.8/9 (2001): 892, 1013, reprinted courtesy of the publisher.

Platt, Frederic. "Waiting" is a section from "The Doctor's Wife Needs an Operation," in *Journal of General Internal Medicine* (1997), reprinted courtesy of the publisher. "Mother Teresa, the Cardiologist," used with permission of the poet.

Powell, Craig. "Poem (Long Overdue) for Mr. Meek" from *I Learn by Going*, South Head Press, 1968, reprinted courtesy of the poet.

Pridmore, Saxby. "New Secure Psychiatric Unit," *Quadrant* (2002), and "The Face," *Studio* (2004), reprinted courtesy of the poet.

Rieves, Dwaine. "Words," *Journal of Medical Humanities* 22.2 (2001): 155–156, and "Gay Men's VD Clinic," *The Lancet* 349 (1997): 1778, reprinted courtesy of the publishers; "Shifts," *Virginia Quarterly Review*, reprinted courtesy of the poet.

Ritchie, Elspeth Cameron. "Gun in the Closet," *Journal of Child and Adolescent Psychopharmacology*, reprinted courtesy of the poet.

Salomon, Bonnie. "Call It," *Journal of Medical Humanities* 23.3/4 (2002): 258–259, reprinted courtesy of the publisher.

Shafer, Audrey. "Loss," *Hiram Poetry Review* 55/56 (1995): 108–109, and "Incompatibility" from *Sleep Talker: Poems by a Doctor/Mother*, Xlibris Press, 2001, reprinted courtesy of the poet; "One Morning," *JAMA* 287.4 (2002): 421, reprinted courtesy of the publisher.

Shen. "Two Men," used with permission of the poet.

Stone, John. "Visitation," "After the Concert: A Confession," and "Transplant" from *Music from Apartment 8: New and Selected Poems*, Louisiana State University Press, 2004, reprinted courtesy of the publisher.

Straus, Marc J. "Sand Crab," "Not God," and "What I Am" from *Symmetry*, Triquarterly Books, Northwestern University Press, 2000, reprinted courtesy of the poet.

Watts, David. "Physical Exam" and "Apnea" from *Taking the History*, Nightshade Press, 1999, reprinted courtesy of the poet; "The Day I Showed My Penis to the Lady Doctor," *Journal of Medical Humanities* 23.3/4 (2002): 260, reprinted courtesy of the publisher.

Weyrauch, Karl. "My Id," *Journal of Medical Humanities* 24.1/2 (2003): 166–167, reprinted courtesy of the publisher; "My Speedometer," *Rosebud* (Fall 2003), reprinted courtesy of the poet.

White, Kelley Jean. "Bleed" from *Late*, People's Press, 2003, and "Kindergarten Physical" from *The Patient Presents*," People's Press, 2001, reprinted courtesy of the poet.

Wintroub, Robert Harlan. "Heart Sounds," *Journal of Medical Humanities* 22.3 (2001): 209, reprinted courtesy of the publisher.

Wright, John. "My Tomography Report," *JAMA* 288.21 (2002) 2651, reprinted courtesy of the publisher. "The Other Man Is Me" and "White Rose," used with permission of the poet.

Young, George. "The Face of Evil," *Annals of Internal Medicine* 133 (2000): 558, reprinted courtesy of the publisher; "Emerson's Aphasia," *Diner*, reprinted courtesy of the poet. "Hutala, Afghanistan," used with permission of the poet.

INDEX OF POEM TITLES